Decision Making in Clinical Surgery

Decision Making in Clinical Surgery

Second Edition

Venkit S Iyer
MBBS MS (Surgery) FACS FRCS(C) FICS
Senior Consultant (Retd)
General and Vascular Surgery
Palm Harbor, Florida, USA

Formerly
Associate Chairman (Surgery)
Jewish Hospital and Medical Center, Brooklyn, New York
Assistant Professor (Surgery)
Albert Einstein College of Medicine, Bronx, New York
Chief (Surgery)
Mease Hospitals, Dunedin and Countryside, Florida
President (Medical Staff)
Helen Ellis Memorial Hospital, Tarpon Springs, Florida, USA
President, North Pinellas Physicians Association
President, Florida Association of Physicians of Indian Origin

Forewords
Muthukumar Muthusamy
Kedambady P Sheka

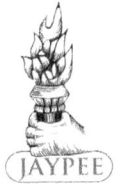

JAYPEE BROTHERS MEDICAL PUBLISHERS
The Health Sciences Publisher
New Delhi | London

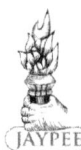
Jaypee Brothers Medical Publishers (P) Ltd.

Headquarters
Jaypee Brothers Medical Publishers (P) Ltd
EMCA House, 23/23-B
Ansari Road, Daryaganj
New Delhi 110 002, India
Landline: +91-11-23272143, +91-11-23272703
+91-11-23282021, +91-11-23245672
Email: jaypee@jaypeebrothers.com

Corporate Office
Jaypee Brothers Medical Publishers (P) Ltd
4838/24, Ansari Road, Daryaganj
New Delhi 110 002, India
Phone: +91-11-43574357
Fax: +91-11-43574314
Email: jaypee@jaypeebrothers.com

Overseas Office
JP Medical Ltd.
83, Victoria Street, London
SW1H 0HW (UK)
Phone: +44 20 3170 8910
Fax: +44 (0)20 3008 6180
Email: info@jpmedpub.com

Website: www.jaypeebrothers.com
Website: www.jaypeedigital.com

© 2024, Jaypee Brothers Medical Publishers

The views and opinions expressed in this book are solely those of the original contributor(s)/author(s) and do not necessarily represent those of editor(s) or publisher of the book.

All rights reserved. No part of this publication may be reproduced, stored or transmitted in any form or by any means, electronic, mechanical, photocopying, recording or otherwise, without the prior permission in writing of the publishers.

All brand names and product names used in this book are trade names, service marks, trademarks or registered trademarks of their respective owners. The publisher is not associated with any product or vendor mentioned in this book.

Medical knowledge and practice change constantly. This book is designed to provide accurate, authoritative information about the subject matter in question. However, readers are advised to check the most current information available on procedures included and check information from the manufacturer of each product to be administered, to verify the recommended dose, formula, method and duration of administration, adverse effects and contraindications. It is the responsibility of the practitioner to take all appropriate safety precautions. Neither the publisher nor the author(s)/editor(s) assume any liability for any injury and/or damage to persons or property arising from or related to use of material in this book.

This book is sold on the understanding that the publisher is not engaged in providing professional medical services. If such advice or services are required, the services of a competent medical professional should be sought.

Every effort has been made where necessary to contact holders of copyright to obtain permission to reproduce copyright material. If any have been inadvertently overlooked, the publisher will be pleased to make the necessary arrangements at the first opportunity.

Inquiries for bulk sales may be solicited at: jaypee@jaypeebrothers.com

Decision Making in Clinical Surgery

First Edition: 2019
Second Edition: **2024**

ISBN: 978-93-5696-268-2

Dedicated to

All my teachers, mentors, and students of surgery.

Foreword

Decision Making in Clinical Surgery by Dr Venkit S Iyer is a very useful guidebook for students of surgery.

Its best value is in getting quick information on day-to-day practice in surgery.

Medical students, Interns, Residents and Junior Surgeons encounter these questions during their rounds, clinics, and operating room all the time.

The language is simple, straightforward and to the point.

Medical science makes steady progress, change is natural. It is up to us to keep up with progress. Learning is a lifelong process. Hence, it is appropriate for the book to be updated periodically, and this second edition is timely.

In this second edition, Dr Iyer has added 10 new chapters and has expanded several of the previous chapters with added information. Several corrections on the previous text have been incorporated.

Information on the use of laparoscopic and robotic instrumentation has been included. New methods in imaging technology that helps surgeons have been mentioned. Advances in endovascular techniques and endoscopic procedures have been included. Safety in surgery has been emphasized. Wound care, infections, intensive care, and interdisciplinary collaboration are some of the topics addressed, in addition to several operative techniques.

Patient presents with a symptom, the doctor encounters a challenge in the operating room, a problem situation is noted in the floor, an urgent situation occurs in the emergency room, a critical condition needs to be handled in the intensive care unit—these are some of the daily encounters in the life of a surgeon. This book gives information on these types of everyday challenges.

I recommend and endorse this second edition.

Muthukumar Muthusamy MD
Chairman
Department of Surgery
South Brooklyn Health
2601 Ocean Parkway
Brooklyn, NY 11235

Foreword

It has been a pleasure for me to review Dr Venkit S Iyer's new improved edition of *Decision Making in Clinical Surgery*. First Edition was well received by the public for whom it was meant. The addition of new chapters such as Infections in Surgery, Carcinoma of Colon and Rectum, Bites and Stings, Surgical Challenges, etc. makes this book a polished work.

Dr Iyer reminds the surgeons not to relinquish the team leadership role of surgeon. Coordinated approach to patient care is the name of the game today. Writers' emphasis is on choosing the right methods, being the patients advocate first and foremost. He reminds us of our serenity prayer: grant me the serenity to accept the things I cannot change, courage to change the things I can, and the wisdom to know the difference.

I wish Dr Iyer's this work will be received well.

Kedambady P Sheka
MD FACS FRCS DABTS
Former Chairman
Surgical Services
Coney Island Hospital
Brooklyn, New York, USA

Preface to the Second Edition

The first edition of this book was published four years ago, as a guide to help students of surgery. Learning is a lifelong process. It helps to have a review book available for quick reference. Standard textbooks are difficult to navigate to find a quick answer for a symptom or a clinical situation.

In this second edition, several of previous chapters have been expanded and updated with current information. In addition, 10 new chapters have been added. Science makes progress and concepts change with time—we must keep up with the information and current thinking.

The theme of the book is a simple approach to clinical situations that the junior surgeons or postgraduate students encounter in daily surgical practice. How to approach a medical complaint by the patient or a problem noticed during rounds or a challenge in the operating room?

The language is simple, direct, and straightforward, just as a senior surgeon will talk to his assistants during rounds or in the operating room. What is the next step, what are the options, what is cost effective, how to make the quickest diagnosis, and how to treat it in the best possible way?

The author sincerely hopes that this book will be useful and valued by medical students, residents and interns, postgraduate students, and junior surgeons.

Venkit S Iyer

Preface to the First Edition

This book is intended to serve as a quick review guide to help medical students, postgraduate students, junior surgeons, or house physicians in clinical practice of surgery. Their daily work is mostly filled with these decision-making issues.

It is not intended to replace any textbooks or treatises in surgery. Topics covered in the book describe a simplistic way to approach surgical problems that will help them in their ordinary work.

The simple format and language will make it user friendly. Emphasis is on common conditions that one encounters in daily rounds or the clinic. Complex conditions and topics are not covered in this book. Complex theories, protocols, and graphics are not described.

The approach is mostly symptom-based and not pathology-based. What is the next step to be taken in a certain situation? What are the most common possibilities? What is most cost effective, what is most expeditious, and what is the quickest way to save lives? How to make a diagnosis, what test is most useful, what procedure is most appropriate? Key steps and techniques involved in several surgical procedures are also discussed.

The author sincerely hopes it will find a place in the personal library of medical students, interns, residents, and young surgeons.

Venkit S Iyer

Acknowledgments

This book is written based on my years of experience and readings. I am grateful to my teachers and mentors over many years. Surgery is both an art and a science, requiring manual dexterity as well as theory knowledge.

I am deeply thankful to Drs Kedambady P Sheka and Muthukumar Muthusamy for reviewing the second edition, making suggestions and writing a Foreword.

I am grateful for the constant support and encouragement of M/s Jaypee Brothers Medical Publishers (P) Ltd, New Delhi, India, in publishing this book. I am extremely thankful to Shri Jitendar P Vij (Group Chairman), Mr Ankit Vij (Managing Director), Mr MS Mani (Group President), Ms Chetna Malhotra (Senior Director—Professional Publishing, Marketing and Business Development), Ms Pooja Bhandari (Director—Production), Mr Anand Kumar and Anirban Mukherjee (Development Editors), who have been prompt, efficient, and helpful.

Contents

SECTION 1: Systemic Topics

1. Process of Decision Making 3
2. Hypotension 4
3. Cardiac Arrhythmia 7
4. Respiratory Distress 9
5. Oliguria 12
6. Fever 14
7. Infections and Surgery 15
8. Antibiotic Therapy 17
9. Nutritional Support 20
10. Electrolytes and Blood Gases 22
11. Multiple Organ Failure 24

SECTION 2: Abdominal Pain

12. Abdominal Pain 29
13. Right Upper Quadrant Abdominal Pain 31
14. Right Lower Quadrant Abdominal Pain 34
15. Left Upper Quadrant Abdominal Pain 36
16. Left Lower Quadrant Abdominal Pain 38
17. Suprapubic Pain 40
18. Mid-Abdominal Pain 41
19. Severe Abdominal Pain 43

SECTION 3: Abdominal Conditions

20. Mass in the Abdomen 47
21. Abdominal Distension 49
22. Abnormal Air 51
23. Back Pain 53
24. Flank Pain 54
25. Jaundice 55
26. Anemia 59
27. Vomiting 61
28. Diarrhea 63
29. Heartburn: Acid Reflux 65
30. Obesity 66
31. Hematemesis 68

SECTION 4: Anorectal Conditions

32. Bleeding Per Rectum 73
33. Pain in the Anal Region 75
34. Hemorrhoids 77
35. Prolapse of the Rectum 79
36. Pruritus Ani 80
37. Pilonidal Cyst 81
38. Carcinoma of Colon and Rectum 82

SECTION 5: Head and Neck

39. Epistaxis 87
40. Mass in Front of the Neck: Thyroid 88
41. Thyroglossal Duct Cyst 91
42. Mass on Side of Neck: Lymph Nodes 92

SECTION 6: Breast

43. Mass in the Breast 97
44. Pain in the Breast 100
45. Bleeding or Discharge from the Nipple 101
46. Gynecomastia 102
47. Abnormal Mammogram 103

SECTION 7: Groin Conditions

48. Mass in the Groin 107
49. Mass in the Scrotum 109
50. Urological Problems in General Surgery 111
51. Hernia 113

SECTION 8: Vascular

52. Varicose Veins 117
53. Swelling of the Legs 119
54. Pain in the Legs 120
55. Numbness of the Legs or Hands 122
56. Gangrene of the Toes 124
57. Ulcerated Leg 127
58. Carotid Artery Surgery 129
59. Abdominal Aortic Aneurysm 132

SECTION 9: Skin and Subcutaneous Tissue

60. Skin Lesions 137
61. Subcutaneous Lumps and Bumps 138

62.	Ganglion Cyst	139
63.	Skin and Subcutaneous Infections	140

SECTION 10: Trauma

64.	Lacerations	145
65.	Stab Wounds	146
66.	Gunshot Wounds	147
67.	Blunt Injuries	148
68.	Blast Injuries	149
69.	Burns	150
70.	Massive External Bleeding	152
71.	Massive Internal Bleeding	154
72.	Bites, Stings, and Scrapes	156

SECTION 11: General Care of Surgical Patient

73.	Preoperative Rounds	161
74.	Postoperative Care	163
75.	Postsurgical Complications	165
76.	Operative Care in General	168
77.	Troubleshooting in the Operating Room	170
78.	Bedside Procedures	172
79.	Cancer Screening	175
80.	What Test, What Method, What Instruments	177
81.	Consultations and Ancillary Services	179
82.	Surgical Challenge Situations	181
83.	Wellness	184
84.	Sign-out and Transfers	186
85.	Safety in Surgery	187
86.	Medical Malpractice Concerns	189

Abbreviations

AAA	:	Abdominal aortic aneurysm		
ABC	:	Airway, breathing, circulation		
AIDS	:	Acquired immunodeficiency syndrome		
Alk. Phos	:	Alkaline phosphatase		
APR	:	Abdominoperineal resection		
ATN	:	Acute tubular necrosis		
BMI	:	Body mass index		
BRCA	:	Breast cancer gene 1 and 2		
BUN	:	Blood urea nitrogen		
Ca	:	Calcium		
CAB	:	Circulation, airway, breathing		
CAT scan	:	Computerized axial tomography scan		
CBC	:	Complete blood count		
CBD	:	Common bile duct		
CCU	:	Coronary care unit		
C-diff	:	*Clostridium difficile*		
Cl	:	Chloride		
CMS	:	Center for Medicare Services		
CO_2	:	Carbon dioxide		
COVID-19	:	Corona virus infection of 2019		
COPD	:	Chronic obstructive pulmonary disease		
CPAP	:	Continuous positive airway pressure		
CPR	:	Cardiopulmonary resuscitation		
CRP	:	C-reactive protein		
CRNA	:	Certified registered nurse anesthetist		
CVP	:	Central venous pressure		
CTA	:	CT angiogram, computerized axial tomography angiogram		
CT Scan	:	Computerized axial tomography scan		
DNA	:	Deoxyribonucleic acid		
DVT	:	Deep vein thrombosis		
DVI	:	Deep vein insufficiency		
EGD	:	Esophagogastroduodenostomy		
EKG	:	Electrocardiogram		
ENT	:	Ear, nose, throat		
ER	:	Emergency room		
ERCP	:	Endoscopic retrograde cholangiopancreatogram		
EVAR	:	Endovascular aortic aneurysm repair		
FAST	:	Focused assessment with sonography for trauma		
FIT test	:	Fecal immunochemical test		
FNA	:	Fine-needle aspiration		
GERD	:	Gastroesophageal reflux disease		
GI	:	Gastrointestinal		
GYN	:	Gynecology		
H_2	:	Hydrogen		
Hb	:	Hemoglobin		
HCT	:	Hematocrit		
HCO_3	:	Bicarbonate		
HER2	:	Human epidermal growth factor 2		
HIDA scan	:	Hepatic iminodiacetic acid scan		
HIV	:	Human immune deficiency virus		
H. pylori	:	*Helicobacter pylori*		
HPV	:	Human papilloma virus		
ICU	:	Intensive care unit		
ID	:	Identification		
IED	:	Improvised explosive device		
IUD	:	Intra Uterine Device		
IV	:	Intravenous		
JCAHO	:	Joint Commission for Accreditation of Hospitals		
K	:	Potassium		
Kg	:	Kilogram		
LFT	:	Liver function test		
LLQ	:	Left lower quadrant		
LUQ	:	Left upper quadrant		
MI	:	Myocardial infarction		
Mg	:	Magnesium		
mg	:	Milligram		
µg	:	Microgram		
MRA	:	Magnetic resonance angiogram		
MRCP	:	Magnetic resonance cholangiopancreatogram		
MRI	:	Magnetic resonance imaging		
MRSA	:	Methicillin-resistant *Staphylococcus aureus*		
Na	:	Sodium		
NG tube	:	Nasogastric tube		
NOTES	:	Natural orifice endoscopic surgery		
NPO	:	Nothing per oral		
O_2	:	Oxygen		
OR	:	Operating room		

PA	:	Physician assistant
PCWP	:	Pulmonary capillary wedge pressure
PE	:	Pulmonary embolism
PEEP	:	Positive end-expiratory pressure
PEG tube	:	Percutaneous endoscopic gastrostomy tube
PIC line	:	Peripherally introduced central line
PID	:	Pelvic inflammatory disease
PPE	:	Personal protective equipment
PPN	:	Peripheral parenteral nutrition
PPH	:	Procedure for prolapsed hemorrhoids
PSA	:	Prostate specific antigen
PT	:	Prothrombin time
PTT	:	Partial thromboplastin time
QI	:	Quality improvement
RAI	:	Radioactive iodine
RBC	:	Red blood cells
RLQ	:	Right lower quadrant
RUQ	:	Right upper quadrant
SCIP	:	Surgical care improvement project
SGOT (AST)	:	Serum glutamic oxaloacetic transaminase
SGPT (ALT)	:	Serum glutamic pyruvic transaminase
SILS	:	Single incision laparoscopic surgery
TAO	:	Thromboangiitis obliterans
TAPP	:	Transabdominal preperitoneal repair
TEM	:	Transrectal endoscopic microsurgery
TEP	:	Total extraperitoneal repair
TIA	:	Transient ischemic attack
TIPS	:	Transjugular intrahepatic portosystemic shunt
TME	:	Total mesorectal excision
TSH	:	Thyroid-stimulating hormone
TPN	:	Total parenteral nutrition
TPA	:	Tissue plasminogen activator
US	:	Ultrasound
US	:	United States
VRE	:	Vancomycin-resistant enterococci
WBC	:	White blood cell

SECTION 1: Systemic Topics

1. Process of Decision Making
2. Hypotension
3. Cardiac Arrhythmia
4. Respiratory Distress
5. Oliguria
6. Fever
7. Infections and Surgery
8. Antibiotic Therapy
9. Nutritional Support
10. Electrolytes and Blood Gases
11. Multiple Organ Failure

CHAPTER 1

Process of Decision Making

INTRODUCTION

You are a young surgeon who has recently completed postgraduate degree course and have full knowledge about surgery. You have a very good theoretical understanding of the subject, are brimming with confidence and optimism, and look forward to a bright future and career. You are young and probably planning to settle down—everything looks good until a real-life test of patient care makes you sweat. Suddenly, you feel so lost and incompetent and wish you had a mentor to guide you. Experience counts, to know what matters, what comes next, and what works best. Decision-making in clinical surgery comes with time and experience.

DECISION-MAKING

Decision-making or "what is the next step" requires theoretical knowledge, clinical acumen, competence, and communication skills. It requires a certain amount of discipline and an understanding of your hospital setup, your community standards, and yourself.

At the bedside, everyone is anxious to know the surgeon's recommendation. Is this patient going to be operated upon? If so, when and where? What type of operation, what are the risks, how much is it going to cost, and will the insurance pay for this procedure? It is a highly charged atmosphere. Surgery is a major decision for the patient as well as for healthcare providers.

It starts with studying the patient chart, talking to the primary care physician, nursing staff, and other relevant healthcare providers. One should review the imaging studies and relevant tests that have been performed before talking to the patient. Now you are armed with maximal information about the patient's condition before walking to the bedside.

Do not forget the basics. A complete history taking and a physical examination consisting of inspection, palpation, percussion, auscultation, and any special examination such as rectal examination or vaginal examination are done while also keeping the patient engaged in a conversation for additional history.

At this point, one should be able to come to a provisional diagnosis. One question I always ask myself is, "Does this patient need immediate surgery as an emergency?" If the answer is "yes," then I move along in that direction. I notify the operating room, anesthesia, and surgical staff to schedule the case and order necessary preoperative workup and preparation. If the patient does not require emergency surgery, then I plan for additional medical treatment, investigation and observation, reevaluation, and a follow-up plan for elective surgery as appropriate. If the patient does not require surgery at all, then I explain the situation and sign off the case.

Decision-making in some of the situations can be straightforward and clearcut. However, in certain other situations, there can be multiple options in the sequence of treatment protocols. Regional and community preferences can be different, due to availability of equipment, cost concerns, cultural differences, education and compliance level of patients, and knowledge base of the surgeons. Even within the same hospital, different surgeons may have different approaches to the same problem.

Practice of surgery is teamwork. It is no longer possible for one single person to manage all aspects of treatment. Obtaining appropriate consultations in a timely manner is part of good decision-making. On the negative side, the healthcare system seems to get fragmented with no leader in-charge of the patient in many instances. It is therefore necessary that the surgeon should always remain in-charge of the patient with a surgical problem to coordinate the care, whether immediate surgery is required or not.

Common things are common. Emphasis is placed on common diagnostic conditions and usual protocols. This book is written with a symptom-based and a clinical care approach rather than going into theory, textbook descriptions, and unusual situations.

CHAPTER 2: Hypotension

INTRODUCTION

Low blood pressure levels need immediate attention in clinical practice. The body is pulling the reserves to maintain its core blood circulation. If left unattended, it will soon lead to catastrophic outcomes, i.e., multisystem failure, and possible death. Shock is a major insult to the tissues at a cellular level, which in turn leads to a series of physiological and pathological changes. Hypotension is one of the clinical manifestations of shock. Shock can be the result of low blood volume as seen in hypovolemic shock, low cardiac output as seen in cardiogenic shock, cell membrane changes as seen in septic shock, anaphylactic reaction, endotoxin insult, and neurological damages, or in multiorgan failures. A quick decision has to be made for the cause of hypotension since corrective steps can be lifesaving.

You are receiving a panic phone call to see a patient who is hypotensive. The patient may be in the emergency department or hospital floor or in the intensive care unit (ICU).

You should immediately go to the location and make personal assessments. There is a tendency to have a prolonged phone conversation with the nurse or junior doctor to obtain the patient's medical history and give instructions. There is nothing wrong with the idea of getting some information and initiating the first-line treatment, but keep it brief and to the point.

The first decision is to find the cause of hypotensive shock. It is divided into three main categories: (1) hypovolemic, (2) cardiogenic, or (3) septic shock. Anaphylactic shock is less common **(Box 2.1)**. The history and physical examination of the patient should help in this case.

BOX 2.1: Types of hypotension shock.
- Hypovolemic → Fluid depletion → Hemorrhagic
- Cardiogenic
- Septic
- Anaphylactic

HYPOTENSIVE SHOCK

Hypovolemic Shock

Hypovolemic shock is suspected from a history of blood loss or fluid loss. Look for internal or external bleeding. External bleeding will be obvious. Internal bleeding can be deceptive. Look for ruptured ectopic pregnancy, ruptured abdominal aneurysms, and blunt injury to the abdomen resulting in splenic laceration, gastrointestinal (GI) bleeding, or bleeding into the chest cavity. When taking the patient's history, ask questions regarding diarrhea and excessive vomiting. Third spacing in acute pancreatitis and sepsis are to be ruled out. Focused assessment with sonography for trauma (FAST) examination is a rapid ultrasound test to detect if there is free fluid, in this case blood in the peritoneal cavity. The same ultrasound probe can be turned upward into the pericardial area to check if there is pericardial tamponade. It is best to avoid wasting valuable time by doing computed tomography (CT) scans.

Treatment requires resuscitation with intravenous (IV) fluids and blood followed by surgery if necessary. The best choice for IV fluid replacement is Ringer's lactate, as it is better to minimize the saline load. Blood loss is replaced with blood transfusion. A 1:1 ratio with packed red blood cells (RBCs) and plasma is used in acute blood loss. Whole blood transfusion is another option.

If there is blood loss, transfer the patient to the operating room as quickly as possible to cease the bleeding. If the hypovolemia is due to fluid loss and not blood loss, then the patient is treated with fluid replacement along with treatment of the underlying cause **(Tables 2.1 and 2.2)**.

Cardiogenic Shock

Cardiogenic shock is suspected with a history of acute chest pain, congestive heart failure, engorged jugulars, chest rales, dyspnea, and a history of cardiac problems, especially in older patients. Request a medical/cardiac consultation,

CHAPTER 2: Hypotension

TABLE 2.1: Causes and treatment of fluid depletion.

Causes	Treatment
Diarrhea	Fluid replacement
Vomiting	Treat underlying cause
Intestinal obstruction	Systemic support
Third spacing in sepsis	Follow-up on labs
Burns	
Pancreatitis	
Poor intake	

TABLE 2.2: Causes and treatment of hemorrhagic shock.

Causes	Treatment
External	
Trauma	Replace blood with blood
Gunshot	IV fluids and blood substitutes
Stab wounds	Stop the bleeding
Falls	Systemic support
Accidents	Follow-up on labs and vital signs
Internal	
Ruptured aneurysms	
Ruptured ectopic pregnancy	
Ruptured spleen	
Accidents	
Trauma	

(IV: Intravenous)

TABLE 2.3: Causes and treatment of septic shock.

Causes	Treatment
Peritonitis	Antibiotics
Ruptured viscus	Remove the focus of sepsis
Perforated appendicitis	IV fluids
Diverticulitis	Surgical corrections
Infected catheters	Systemic support
Urinary sepsis	Follow-up monitoring
Infected implants	
Pneumonia	
Pleural infections	

(IV: Intravenous)

electrocardiogram (EKG), chest X-ray, and cardiac enzymes. Avoid fluid overload.

In cases of trauma associated with cardiogenic shock, one must think of pericardial tamponade, myocardial contusion or injury, air embolism, or tension pneumothorax. In young patients with a history of injury to the chest wall, one should entertain a high index of suspicion of the above and perform quick needle aspirations or a chest X-ray to confirm or treat the above entities.

Septic Shock

Septic shock is suspected with a history of fever, recent GI surgery, urinary tract infections, soft-tissue infections, and pelvic infections. Examination may reveal peritonitis and tense and tender abdomen **(Table 2.3)**. Other causes of sepsis include line-related sepsis, such as infected catheters, ports or grafts, and endocarditis.

Treatment is using appropriate antibiotic coverage, usually broad-spectrum, and fluid replacement to maintain adequate preload. The patient may require a large amount of fluid due to low afterload and capillary leak due to endotoxin. Watch for oliguria. The most important step is to eliminate the focus of sepsis. This may require removal of infected catheter, drainage of pus or empyema, or laparotomy to remove a ruptured appendix or perforated colon, as the case dictates.

PRACTICAL STEPS IN MANAGING PATIENTS WITH HYPOTENSION

Irrespective of the cause of hypotension and the type of shock, all patients are monitored and tested initially in a similar way. Exact treatment might vary depending upon the etiology.

First Step

In order to monitor the patient in the acute care setting, one would set up an EKG monitor on the digital screen, have an automatic blood pressure recording that reads the blood pressure every so often, and a pulse oximetry that measures oxygen saturation. A Foley catheter is inserted to measure urine output. An intravenous line is set up for administration of fluids and medications. Body temperature, clinical sensorium, and neurological status are recorded, and a flowchart is initiated showing frequent vital signs and hourly intake and output. The blood sample is sent for complete blood count, basic metabolic profile, and any additional tests depending upon the underlying diagnosis. If hemorrhagic shock is in consideration, blood is sent for type and crossmatch; if cardiac condition is in consideration, blood is sent for cardiac enzymes, and in abdominal conditions amylase and lipase are requested.

Further Monitoring

Central line placement: This is a useful step, since one can measure the central venous pressure (CVP) and at the same time ensure reliable central intravenous access with three lumens for administration of fluids, blood, medications and nutrients. CVP is low in hypovolemic shock and needs rapid infusion of fluids or blood if necessary. It can be high in cardiogenic shock. In septic shock, it can be variable depending upon the intravascular filling pressure.

Arterial line placement: This is done in selected situations, when the blood pressure measurement by a regular manometer is unreliable, or if the patient is going to be intubated and be on a ventilator for a period of time. It will also be useful if the patient is to undergo major surgery or requires frequent blood gas monitoring.

Swan-Ganz catheter placement: This is a useful step for continued care of the patient in the ICU. It measures the left heart filling pressure by pulmonary artery wedge pressure (PCWP), provides mixed venous oxygen measurement, and provides cardiac output measurement. These values are useful in titrating the fluid replacement and avoiding pulmonary edema and managing fluctuating cardiorespiratory status and fluid replacement. In septic shock, the patient may look edematous and bloated due to capillary leak, but the intravascular volume can be low. PCWP and cardiac output measurements are valuable guides in these critically ill patients.

Medications

Various medications are considered for bringing up the blood pressure, mainly with the goal of maintaining renal perfusion, to reduce chance of renal shutdown. Medications are adjuncts to primary treatment with fluid replacement and correcting the underlying cause.

- *For hypotension:*
  - *Dopamine:* 1-1.5 µg/kg/min infusion
  - *Levophed:* 4 mg in 1,000 mL of dextrose titrated to keep blood pressure 80 systolic
  - *Dobutamine:* 0.5-1 µg/kg/min
- *For infections and septic shock:* Broad spectrum antibiotics.
- *For anaphylactic shock:* Epinephrine, 0.5-0.1 mg IV.
- *For cardiogenic shock:* Medications based on cardiology recommendations
- *Medications to avoid in the initial stages of assessment:* Diuretics, sedatives, bicarbonates, and steroids

IV Solutions

- Start with Ringer's lactate or normal saline.
- Blood loss is replaced with blood—use whole blood if available. If components are used, give packed cell, plasma, and platelets in a 1:1:1 ratio.
- If colloids are used, consider hydroxyethyl starch, dextran, or albumin.

KEY POINTS

It is important for the surgeon to recognize volume depletion and sepsis. Start IV fluids, correct the cause of hypotension, and provide emergency care.

CHAPTER 3: Cardiac Arrhythmia

INTRODUCTION

All physicians and nurses should know how to perform a cardiopulmonary resuscitation (CPR) in case of an emergency. It can happen anywhere in the hospital and sometimes in public places. One should check for a pulse by feeling the carotid artery and check for breathing. The old dictum of airway, breathing, and circulation known as ABC, the sequence in which one conducted the CPR in the past, has been currently modified as circulation, airway, and breathing (CAB) in that sequence to conduct the CPR. In other words, one would start chest compressions first, as soon as the absence of carotid pulse is discovered. After about 20 chest compressions, the airway is checked and assisted breathing is started. After four quick breaths, chest compression is resumed and the cardiac rhythm is checked. Further interventions depend on the cardiac status.

ARRHYTHMIAS

This topic is usually for the medical and cardiology students. However, surgery students should also know the fundamentals and be able to handle emergency situations. Advanced cardiac life support (ACLS) and advanced trauma life support (ATLS) are integral parts of the course on trauma and critical care. All physicians should know how to recognize common arrhythmias, start urgent treatments, or conduct CPR.

- Sinus tachycardia
- Sinus bradycardia
- Paroxysmal atrial tachycardia
- Atrial fibrillation
- Ventricular tachycardia
- Ventricular fibrillation
- Heart blocks—first degree, second degree, and third degree
- Premature ventricular contractions
- Agonal rhythm and asystole.

Common types of arrhythmias have been described in **Figures 3.1 to 3.10**.

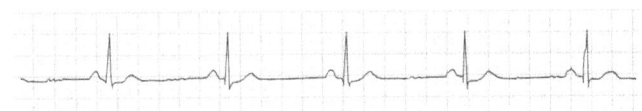

Fig. 3.1: Sinus bradycardia.
- Does not require any treatment most of the time.
- Rule out causation by beta blockers or other drugs.
- May need atropine at times.

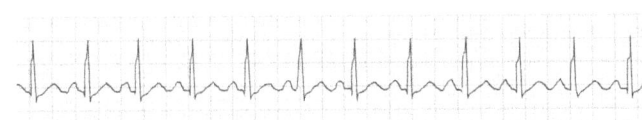

Fig. 3.2: Sinus tachycardia.
- Cause could include hypovolemia, sepsis, hemorrhage, pain, exercise, stress, and shock of any type.
- Treat the underlying cause.
- May need fluid replacement, blood, antibiotics, pain medications, and drugs as needed.

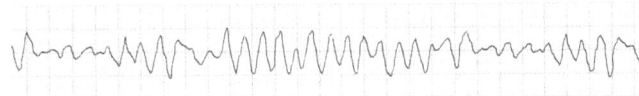

Fig. 3.3: Ventricular fibrillation.
- Needs immediate defibrillation followed by full CPR.
- May be having myocardial infarction.

(CPR: cardiopulmonary resuscitation)

SECTION 1: Systemic Topics

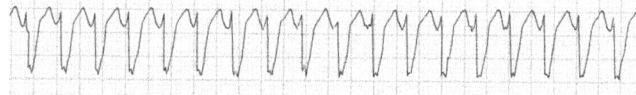

Fig. 3.4: Ventricular tachycardia.
- Initiate CPR measures.
- Amiodarone IV.

(CPR: cardiopulmonary resuscitation; IV: intravenous)

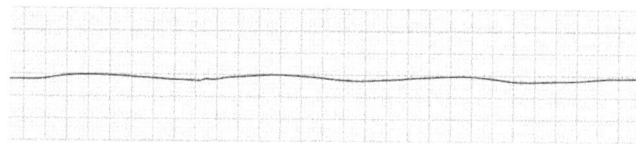

Fig. 3.5: Asystole (cardiac arrest rhythm).
- Initiate CPR measures.
- Epinephrine IV or intracardiac.

(CPR: cardiopulmonary resuscitation; IV: intravenous)

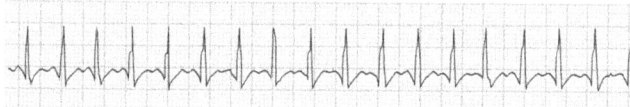

Fig. 3.6: Supraventricular tachycardia.
- Treatment needed.
- Adenosine, diltiazem, verapamil.

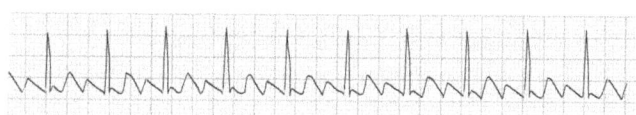

Fig. 3.7: Atrial flutter.
- Diltiazem to control ventricular rate.
- Ablation.
- Anticoagulation.

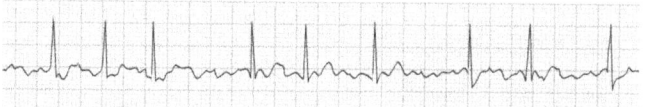

Fig. 3.8: Atrial fibrillation.
- Diltiazem to control ventricular rate.
- Ablation.
- Anticoagulation.

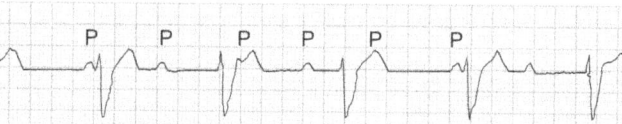

Fig. 3.9: Third-degree heart block.
- External pacing in monitored bed.
- Temporary pacemaker followed by permanent pacemaker.

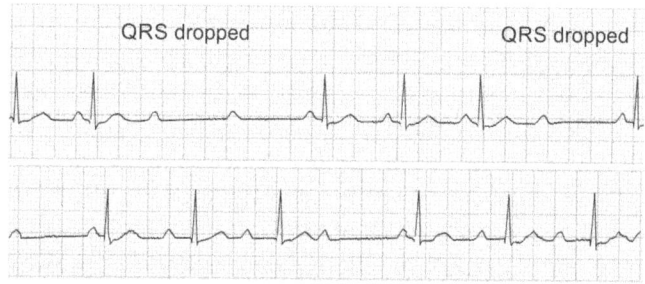

Fig. 3.10: Second-degree heart block.
- Permanent pacemaker.

KEY POINTS

All physicians should be able to recognize common cardiac arrhythmias and take emergency steps to treat them. Obviously, a subsequent cardiology consultation will be requested for proper remedy.

CHAPTER 4

Respiratory Distress

INTRODUCTION

Airway and breathing management is the basic step in saving lives. Management of any ill patient will need assessment of ventilation equilibrium, with reference to oxygen saturation as well as carbon dioxide exchange. Sometimes, quick decisions have to be made to remove objects blocking the upper airway and to establish a clear air passage. Moreover, it may require a slow and careful assessment of the acid–base metabolic balance and adjustments on the ventilator. A patient may be having labored breathing from a tension pneumothorax or from congestive heart failure. How does one make quick decisions? What test to order? What interventions would be best?

MANAGEMENT (TABLES 4.1 AND 4.2)

The patient cannot breathe. You are called to the bedside STAT. What can you do?

Do not panic and cause more commotion. There are probably some caregivers already at the bedside, ready to give some information. Get the history while making observations at the same time.

Does this patient need an immediate airway access? Is this a time for emergency cricothyroid needle puncture or an emergency on the spot tracheostomy? Is this a case for Heimlich maneuver due to food bolus in the throat? Is the patient awake and breathing? Does this patient need emergency endotracheal intubation? Can you just give oxygen with a facemask or do you need an Ambu' bag? All these questions keep swirling your mind in a second.

Open the patient's mouth and inspect the nasal and oral airways. Check to inspect if anything is blocking the passages, such as blood, foreign bodies, food bolus, vomitus, or an edematous tongue.

Does the patient need urgent endotracheal intubation? Can you give adequate ventilation with the facemask and oxygen? What does the pulse oximetry show about the oxygen saturation level? What is the rhythm on cardiac monitoring?

Auscultate the lungs. Are breath sounds equal and audible, or are there crepitus and rhonchi? Is there a tension pneumothorax, collapse of the lung, or massive pleural fluid collection? Is the patient blue and cyanotic or is this a pink puffer? Are there obvious moist rales and rhonchi with crepitus sounds? Is there severe bronchospasm? Is there evidence of surgical emphysema with a crackling soap bubble-type feel under the skin?

TABLE 4.1: Causes of respiratory distress

Upper airway	Lower airway	Chest wall	Central nervous
Facial trauma	Bronchial asthma	Fracture of ribs	Drug overdose
Neck injury	Congestive heart failure	Pneumothorax	Toxemia
Food bolus	Pneumonia	Hemothorax	Head injury
Blood and vomitus	Pulmonary embolism	Empyema	Spinal cord injury
Laryngeal pathology	Collapse of lung	Consolidation	Brain tumors
Carcinoma	Pulmonary congestion	Trapped lung	Encephalopathy
Aspiration	ARDS		Medications
Drowning			

(ARDS: acute respiratory distress syndrome)

Ask for an emergency portable chest X-ray and look for pneumothorax, hemothorax, consolidation or collapse of one lung, pneumonia, or congestive heart failure.

If evidence of tension pneumothorax is noted, one can immediately insert a large-bore needle along the midclavicular line at the second or third intercostal space, followed by insertion of a small-sized cannula loaded on a needle 6–12F (pigtail catheter kit), or if time permits insertion of a chest tube 20–30F. These tubes are then connected to an underwater seal or to a one-way valve application (Heimlich flutter valve). This will allow the lung to expand immediately. Spontaneous pneumothorax is often due to ruptured emphysematous bullae on the lung surface. If the air leak persists beyond a 1-week time following pneumothorax from any etiology, the patient may need surgical intervention.

If there is evidence of a massive pleural effusion or a hemothorax, one should tap the sixth intercostal space with a large-bore needle to confirm the same, and then replace it with a chest tube connected to an underwater seal.

If there is evidence of total collapse of the lung due to a blocking agent in the bronchial stem, such as a foreign body or mucous plug, immediate arrangements are made for bronchoscopic aspiration or retrieval.

An immediate decision is made at the bedside as to how to establish the airway, how to provide adequate oxygenation, and how to then treat the underlying medical problem that led to this state **(Fig. 4.1)**.

Start with a tight facemask and oxygen. Insert an airway, either orally or nasally, at the same time. If there is any question about satisfactory progress, immediately perform endotracheal intubation and place the patient on mechanical ventilation **(Fig. 4.2)**.

TABLE 4.2: Diagnosis and treatment of respiratory distress

Diagnosis	Treatment
Inspect upper airway	Remove obstructing materials in oral cavity
Inspect oral cavity	Mask ventilation (Ambu® bag)
Listen for breath sounds	Endotracheal intubation
Evaluate neurological status	Cricothyroidotomy
Chest X-ray	Tracheostomy
CT scan	Treat the underlying cause
	Ventilator support

(CT: computed tomography)

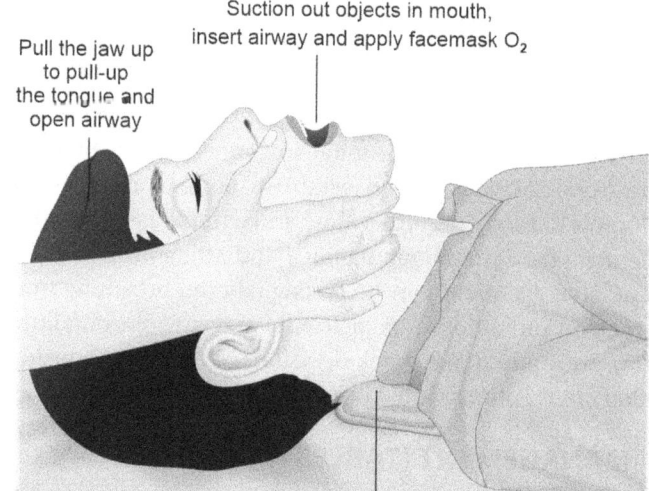

Fig. 4.1: Emergency airway management.

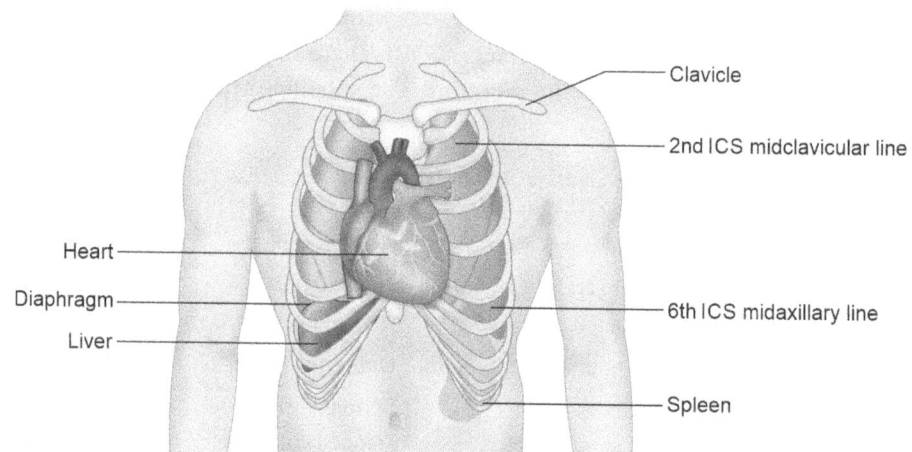

Fig. 4.2: Safe places to insert chest tube or needle aspiration—2nd intercostal space (ICS) midclavicular line or 6th ICS midaxillary line.

If this is a patient who is to be taken to an operating room soon for an underlying problem such as trauma or a gunshot wound, one might as well intubate the patient in the emergency room (ER) and be ready.

If this is a patient with congestive heart failure, one may give a facemask and oxygen and follow the patient in the coronary care unit (CCU) while being medically managed with diuretics and cardiac medications.

The issue of central nervous system depressants inducing respiratory suppression needs to be evaluated and addressed. Very often, we see this in the recovery room after surgery and anesthesia. The patient has not fully recovered and awakened from anesthesia or is oversedated. Sometimes, the patient has taken an overdose of addictive drugs such as heroin, cocaine, morphine, or fentanyl. Sometimes, it is an after effect of brain injury, spinal cord injury, or advanced toxemia related to hepatic failure, renal failure, or poisoning. These patients have very shallow breathing at a slow rate. Pulse oximetry may show low oxygen saturation along with blood gases showing severe respiratory acidosis. The patients are not responsive to questioning or to awakening methods. The patients just look too sleepy.

Medications of use are respiratory stimulants such as doxapram or antidotes to morphine such as Narcan® (naloxone), and thiamine for encephalopathy.

KEY POINTS

First, make sure that the airway is good and is secured. Then correct the disease process while providing ventilator assistance.

CHAPTER 5

Oliguria

INTRODUCTION

A low urine output is a warning sign of impending renal problems and can be corrected if timely action is taken. For the surgeons, it is important to recognize hypovolemia and begin administration of IV fluids and transfusion of blood or blood substitutes before acute renal failure (ARF) or acute tubular necrosis (ATN) settles. Use of diuretics such as Lasix® at this phase will further deplete the blood volume and expedite the onset of ATN. It is also important to recognize nephrotoxic medications and antibiotics and avoid them on patients with marginal renal function. Prerenal, renal, and postrenal causes of renal failure have to be kept in mind and ruled out in a systematic manner. Early nephrology consultation and dialysis can offset permanent renal failure in many instances.

CASE AND MANAGEMENT

"Doctor, the urine output has been low for the past several hours." the nurse reports during the rounds.

If there is no Foley catheter, insert a Foley. If there is a catheter already in place, check and make sure that it is patent and not clogged or kinked.

Now check the chart and review intake and output records, history, and examination of the patient. What was the diagnosis at the time of admission, what has been done, what medications have been administered, and what has been the progress so far?

There is a tendency to give Lasix® initially. Hold the urge. Hold diuretics until you have made a good assessment of the cause of oliguria **(Table 5.1)**.

Is there a reason for this patient to be hypovolemic? If so, a fluid challenge with 500 mL of normal saline over 30 minutes would be appropriate. The patient may be dehydrated on examination and lacking in fluid intake on chart review, which makes it easy to follow-up on fluid challenge with more IV fluids.

TABLE 5.1: Causes of oliguria.

Prerenal	Renal	Postrenal
Hypovolemia	Acute nephritis	Hydronephrosis
Hemorrhagic shock	Chronic nephritis	Congenital issues
Septic shock	Drug induced	Polycystic kidney
Acute pancreatitis	Sepsis	Bladder neck obstruction
Major trauma	Autoimmune	Ureteric stones
Dehydration	Toxemia	Prostate problems
Congestive failure	Anaphylactic	Renal tumors
Cardiogenic shock		Trauma
		Retroperitoneal fibrosis

The patient may be having hypoperfusion due to congestive heart failure, with edematous soft tissues. In this situation, one may want to use diuretics in moderation while maintaining an adequate perfusion pressure.

The patient could be in septic shock with swollen soft tissues due to third spacing. This is a tricky situation that requires further monitoring such as central venous pressure (CVP) or Swan–Ganz catheter to monitor the filling pressure. The patients may look well hydrated but may actually need more volume administration to maintain the filling pressure before using small doses of diuretics.

The patient could go into ATN or acute renal failure due to the underlying disorder. This also requires judicious use of diuretics, IV fluids, and close monitoring. A rapid rise of blood urea nitrogen (BUN) and creatinine with persistent oliguria warrants a nephrology consultation. Problems related to the urinary tract such as obstruction of bladder, ureters, and kidneys might require a urology consultation.

A nephrology consultation is requested if renal failure appears to be imminent. Prepare for long-term or short-term hemodialysis. In many instances, a few sittings of temporary hemodialysis would be adequate. Given time, the renal

> **BOX 5.1:** Treatment of oliguria.
> - Insert Foley catheter if not in place already
> - Check Foley for blocks and kinks
> - Fluid challenge if hypovolemia is suspected
> - Treat the underlying cause
> - Judicious use of diuretics
> - Hydration and blood transfusion as needed
> - Temporary hemodialysis
> - Plan for long-term hemodialysis
> - Correct metabolic problems

function may recover. This is especially true in acute sepsis that has been corrected or in acute pancreatitis, poisoning, or trauma cases. The surgeon may be requested to insert temporary dialysis catheters. It can be done at the bedside or in the operating room with help of fluoroscopy. It can be inserted via the subclavian vein, internal jugular vein, or femoral vein routes.

Correct electrolyte abnormalities involving Na, K, Mg, Ca, and HCO—one must watch for hyperkalemia and acidosis **(Box 5.1)**. Maintain nutritional support and provide metabolic support. Avoid nephrotoxic drugs.

KEY POINTS

Resist the use of Lasix® when you hear about oliguria and find the cause of oliguria. Fluid challenge is the first-line therapy when hypovolemia is suspected.

CHAPTER 6

Fever

INTRODUCTION

For the surgeon, fever is a symptom of a more serious underlying infection. Hence, the priority should be to find the cause of fever and treat the same, while efforts are made to reduce the body temperature.

DISCUSSION

Fever is one of the most common symptoms noticed by the patient and nursing staff while they are taking the vital signs. A temperature chart is displayed at the bedside showing a graphic pattern visible to the caregivers. A daily spike in the temperature chart is a challenge for the doctor.

A systematic evaluation of the patient by taking history and physical examination is needed. The focus is to find the cause of fever. When a patient is admitted to the hospital with fever, it could be related to a surgical pathology or a nonsurgical problem.

Most commonly, a new admission with fever is due to nonsurgical infectious conditions such as COVID-19, or other viral infections, bacterial infections, urinary tract infections, pulmonary infections, endocarditis, or other rare conditions. They could also have surgically correctable pathologies such as ascending cholangitis, acute cholecystitis, acute appendicitis, peritonitis from various reasons, acute diverticulitis, pelvic inflammatory disease, acute pyelonephritis, infected grafts or catheters, or deep-seated abscesses.

If this happens to be a postsurgical patient, one will think of wound infection, atelectasis of lung, infected intravenous lines or urinary catheters, intra-abdominal infections, or infected implanted devices such as grafts, ports, or pumps.

Tests are done to aid the diagnosis which includes complete blood count, cultures of blood, wound, drainage fluid, and urine. X-ray of chest is taken.

Treatment involves removal of the source of infection as soon as possible. This includes inspection of all wounds, opening of suspected wound infections, and drainage of abscesses. The patient is ambulated and pulmonary toilet is attended to. Urinary catheter and intravenous (IV) lines are removed as soon as feasible. Infected grafts, devices, and catheters are removed. Abscesses are drained and inflamed organs such as the gallbladder and appendix are removed. Antibiotics are started based on the most educated guess of the organism and modified as and when culture and sensitivity results come back. In the meantime, efforts are made to reduce the body temperature with the use of aspirin or paracetamol, and cold tepid sponges.

KEY POINTS

Fever is a manifestation of an underlying infection. Efforts are made to identify the source of infection and remove it, along with antibiotic therapy and temperature control.

CHAPTER 7

Infections and Surgery

INTRODUCTION

Infections are nightmares for the surgeon. They can happen following surgery, but every effort must be made to reduce surgical site infections (SSI) especially after elective surgery. Certain infections require surgery for correction.

CATEGORIES OF CASES

Surgical procedures can be classified as clean cases, clean contaminated cases, contaminated cases, or grossly contaminated cases.

Clean cases are elective procedures, where there was no infection to start with. Examples of such surgery would include elective hernia repair, placement of pacemaker, or excision of a breast mass. These wounds should not get infected. Causes of such an infection are contamination of the wound, poor aseptic precautions, poor sterilization of instruments, or preexisting unrecognized infection in the patient. As prophylaxis, one dose of antibiotic of first-generation cephalosporin or similar antibiotic is administered 1 hour before the incision time by the intravenous route. No further antibiotics are needed for such cases.

Clean contaminated cases are elective procedures involving organs that have bacterial flora and stand a chance to get infected, especially if there is a spillage during the procedure. Examples of such procedures are elective cholecystectomy, elective gastric surgery, surgery in the oral cavity, anal procedures, or nasal procedures. They are given a prophylactic antibiotic for the first 24 hours and stopped. The wounds can be closed primarily.

Contaminated cases are already infected to start with and carry a higher chance for postoperative infection of the wound and abscess formation. Examples of such cases are acute cholecystitis, perforated acute appendicitis, acute diverticulitis, or necrotizing soft-tissue infections. These patients need prophylactic and therapeutic antibiotic coverage for 1 week. These wounds should be left open partially or fully and covered with light moist dressings.

Grossly contaminated cases are obviously and grossly infected. Examples are perforated viscus with gross peritonitis, compound fracture following a street accident, gas gangrene, and patients in septic shock. These patients should receive broad-spectrum antibiotic coverage from the time of diagnosis till the end of the infectious process. Wounds are totally left open for secondary closure afterward.

DRAINS

Usage of drains is to be decided based on the type of infection and chances of continued leakage following the surgical procedure. Drains will reduce the chances of postoperative infection and fluid collection at the site of surgery and can be lifesaving in certain situations. They are placed following radical mastectomy, radical lymph node dissections, following surgery for acute cholecystitis, when bile leakage is a consideration, following duodenal surgery, following low anterior resection, or following drainage of various abscess. Whenever possible, closed suction drainage is preferred for better follow-up care, measurement of drainage amount, and patient comfort.

The drainage fluid is inspected, measured, and cultured if necessary. The time to remove a drain tube is when it is no longer serving a function and not set by a certain time period. For example, a postcholecystectomy drain with bile content in it is left in place until definitive treatment is completed, and the bile leakage has stopped.

PREVENTION OF SURGICAL SITE INFECTION

Efforts to reduce SSI should start from the outpatient setting or from the initial office visit. Those who are heavy smokers, markedly obese, diabetics, malnourished, and immunocompromised or on certain medications such as steroids are at a higher risk for wound infection, and poor tissue healing. These risk factors should be corrected as best as possible before scheduling elective surgery.

In the preoperative stage, one should look for lung infections, urinary tract infections, and skin infections. These items should be treated first and surgery postponed if necessary.

Surgery site preparation is better done with clippers, just before the procedure instead of shaving the night before. Washing the site with soap and water and cleansing with chlorhexidine sponges are done before draping. Swiping the exposed areas with alcohol and using Steri-Drapes will further protect the skin.

During surgery, efforts must be made to minimize tissue dissections, avoid spillage or contamination from internal organs, reduce bleeding and hematoma formation, isolate clean areas from contaminated areas, and minimize the operating time. Good surgical techniques, knowledge of the anatomy, and tissue handling are important factors. If every step is done right with a plan and purpose, the procedure goes smooth, in a timely fashion.

COVID-19 AND SURGERY

The pandemic COVID-19 caused great havoc across the globe with millions killed and disabled in a short span of time. Lessons learned are good for the future, and are still being followed, even if the pandemic appears to be in control.

All patients should be asked about symptoms of fever, cough, and respiratory problems before scheduling elective surgery. If there is any suspicion, a rapid COVID test should be done and if positive, elective surgery should be postponed until it is cleared.

Personal protective equipment with masks, gloves, gowns, and drapes should be used by all providers and by the patient. Isolation precautions, minimizing the number of personnel in the operating room, enhanced cleansing and disinfectants, less use of electrocautery, nebulizers, enhanced smoke control to limit aerosolization, and reducing personal contacts by using telemedicine are ways to reduce the risk for the caregivers as well as the patient.

KEY POINTS

All efforts should be made to reduce SSI. Attention to details from the office visit to the postoperative phase is needed.

CHAPTER 8

Antibiotic Therapy

INTRODUCTION

Antibiotics are cornerstones of surgery in modern practice. Infections were rampant before the antibiotic era. Many serious infections ended up in mortality. Surgical complications were high. Pus was called "laudable" since it meant that the infection is contained and can be drained. The problem we are facing today is the overabundance of antibiotics and abuse of the same, resulting in adverse drug reactions and serious side effects as well as development of antibiotic resistance to bacteria. Prophylactic antibiotics are used as protection against compromise in sterility and technical perfection. There must be a reason for the use of a certain antibiotic either by proven culture and sensitivity or by evidence-based medicine.

A very common question during the rounds is to decide whether the patient should be given antibiotics or not. If so, what medication, what dose, and for how long? Cost concerns along with quality concerns make this an often confusing topic, with different individuals taking different approaches.

However, certain generalities are well accepted. Antibiotics are given either prophylactic or therapeutic regimens. Prophylactic antibiotics are used only sparingly and for short periods of time.

ANTIBIOTICS

All elective surgical procedures receive a single dose of antibiotic given within 1 hour before the incision, irrespective of the nature of the surgery. The choice depends on the patient's drug allergy and coexisting conditions. Generally speaking, a first-generation cephalosporin would be adequate. If there is a cardiac issue such as prior valve replacement, an additional dosage of vancomycin or clindamycin may be needed.

If it is a clean case, no further administration of antibiotic is needed (e.g., hernia repair). If this is a clean contaminated case, then the antibiotics are continued for 24 hours and stopped (e.g., acute appendicitis without perforation removed with no contamination, elective colon resection). If it is a grossly infected case, then antibiotics are given for a full course of 7 days (e.g., perforated diverticulitis).

Therapeutic antibiotic administration is for obviously infected cases. The choice of antibiotic depends on culture, sensitivity, and anticipated spectrum of contamination based on clinical judgment. Certain conditions such as bacterial endocarditis, infected joints, infected implants, and infected grafts may need several weeks of therapy. In these cases, consultation with an infectious disease consultant would be helpful. In treating grossly infected situations, broad-spectrum coverage will be needed, often combining third-generation cephalosporins with aminoglycosides and antibacterial (e.g. Zosyn®, gentamicin, and Flagyl®) and antifungal (e.g. Diflucan®) agents.

Special situations—methicillin-resistant *Staphylococcus aureus* (MRSA), vancomycin-resistant enterococci (VRE), *Clostridium difficile* (*C. difficile*), and fungal infections—may arise where patients would need further care with isolation, cross-contamination precautions, and additional special prescription medications.

It is a general observation that there is abuse of antibiotics in many instances. Antibiotics are either unnecessary, used for prolonged periods of time, or used indiscriminately without reason. This is a costly habit with many side effects. Resistance to antibiotics develops with the evolution of drug-resistant bacteria. It also leads to allergic reactions and

---

BOX 8.1: Aminoglycosides.

- Amikacin—for gram-negative bacteria
- Gentamicin—*Escherichia coli*
- Kanamycin—*Klebsiella*
- Neomycin—*Pseudomonas aeruginosa*
- Tobramycin—for gram-negative bacteria

conditions such as *C. difficile* colitis. Every antibiotic ordered should have a scientific justification based on culture and sensitivity, observed infection, or evidence-based studies.

A list of commonly used antibiotics and bacterial effectiveness is given in **Boxes 8.1 to 8.13**. Dosage depends on different factors.

BOX 8.2: Carbapenems.

- Broad-spectrum coverage, against both gram positives and negatives
- Ertapenem (Invanz®)
- Doripenem (Doribax®)
- Imipenem/cilastatin (Primaxin®)
- Meropenem (Merrem®)

BOX 8.3: First-generation cephalosporins.

- Good for gram-positive infections
- Cefadroxil (Duricef®)
- Cefazolin (Ancef®)
- Cefalotin (Keflin®)
- Cefalexin (Keflex®)

BOX 8.4: Third-generation cephalosporins.

- Gram-positive coverage and gram-negative coverage, except *Pseudomonas*
- Ceftazidime (Fortaz®)
- Ceftriaxone (Rocephin®)
- Cefotaxime (Claforan®)

BOX 8.5: Penicillins.

- Wide range of infections, streptococci, gram positives, spirochetes, Lyme disease
- Amoxicillin
- Ampicillin
- Dicloxacillin
- Methicillin
- Nafcillin
- Penicillin G
- Ticarcillin

BOX 8.6: Penicillin combinations.

- Broad-spectrum coverage
- Amoxicillin/Clavulanate (Augmentin®)
- Ampicillin/Sulbactam (Unasyn®)
- Piperacillin/Tazobactam (Zosyn®)
- Ticarcillin/Clavulanate (Timentin®)

BOX 8.7: Antibiotics used for methicillin-resistant *Staphylococcus aureus* (MRSA).

- Clindamycin (Cleocin®)
- Vancomycin
- Linezolid (Zyvox®)
- Daptomycin
- Doxycycline
- Tigecycline
- Delafloxacin (Baxdela®)

BOX 8.8: Antibiotics used for tuberculosis.

- Streptomycin
- Rifampin (Rifadin®)
- Ethambutol
- Isoniazid (INH®)
- Pyrazinamide (Aldinamide®)
- Cycloserine (Seromycin®)
- Rifapentine (Priftin®)
- Capreomycin (Capastat®)

BOX 8.9: Antibiotics used for streptococcal infections.

- Also useful for upper respiratory infections and lower respiratory infections
- Azithromycin (Zithromax®)
- Clarithromycin (Biaxin®)
- Erythromycin (Erythrocin®)
- Roxithromycin
- Daptomycin (Cubicin®)

BOX 8.10: Other antibiotics used for important diseases.

- Antifungal—Fluconazole (Diflucan), Amphotericin
- For *Clostridium difficile*—Vancomycin, Metronidazole (Flagyl®), Fidaxomycin
- For leprosy—Dapsone, Clofazimine
- For bowel preparation—Neomycin, erythromycin
- For urinary tract infections—Ciprofloxacin, Bactrim, Nitrofurantoin (Macrodantin®)
- For typhoid, cholera, and typhus—Chloramphenicol

BOX 8.11: Broad-spectrum synthetic antibiotics.

- Antihelminths—Furazolidone (Furoxone®), albendazole, mebendazole
- Quinolones—for GI infections, urinary infections, pneumonia—Ciprofloxacin (Cipro), Gatifloxacin (Tequin), Levofloxacin (Levaquin)
- Azactam (aztreonam)—for gram negatives
- Sulfa drugs—Sulfadiazine, Sulfisoxazole (Gantrisin), Sulfamethizole (Thiosulfil Forte), Trimethoprim–Sulfamethoxazole (Bactrim)—for urinary infections, eye infections

(GI: gastrointestinal)

BOX 8.12: Skin infections and topical agents.

- Mafenide (Sulfamylon®)
- Silver sulfadiazine (Silvadene®)
- Neosporin
- Bacitracin

BOX 8.13: Drugs used for HIV/AIDS—antivirals.

- Abacavir (Ziagen®)
- Didanosine (Videx®)
- Emtricitabine (Emtriva®)
- Lamivudine (Epivir®)
- Stavudine (Zerit®)
- Tenofovir (Viread®)
- Zidovudine (Retrovir®)
- Efavirenz (Sustiva®)
- Etravirine (Intelence®)
- Nevirapine (Viramune®)
- Rilpivirine (Edurant®)
- Atazanavir (Reyataz®)
- Darunavir (Prezista®)
- Fosamprenavir (Lexiva®)
- Indinavir (Crixivan®)
- Nelfinavir (Viracept®)
- Ritonavir (Norvir®)
- Enfuvirtide (Fuzeon®)
- Maraviroc (Selzentry®)
- Dolutegravir (Tivicay®)
- Raltegravir (Isentress®)
- Cobicistat (Tybost®)

(AIDS: acquired immune deficiency syndrome; HIV: human immunodeficiency virus)

KEY POINTS

Do not prescribe antibiotics indiscriminately. Stop them once the immediate use is over. A single dose of antibiotics within an hour before surgery is all that is needed for surgical prophylaxis.

CHAPTER 9

Nutritional Support

INTRODUCTION

For a good recovery following surgery or a major illness, one must pay attention to the good nutritional status of the patient. Anergy is the term used when the patient just does not thrive. Surgery is a major trauma to the body. Serious illness and trauma demand higher metabolic support; moreover, the patient is already starving or chronically depleted to start with. Any patient who is likely to starve for more than 1 week should be started on a nutritional supplement program. Enteral alimentation is the first preference for nutritional support for those who can use their gastrointestinal (GI) tract **(Table 9.1)**. For all others, parenteral support in the form of total parenteral nutrition (TPN) or peripheral parenteral nutrition (PPN) is ordered **(Table 9.2)**. Calculation of fluid volume, calories, and components along with supplemental addition of vitamins and trace elements is taken into consideration while ordering the TPN formula.

ASSESSMENT

Assessment of nutritional status and nutritional needs is an integral part of routine patient care.

All patients who are likely to be starving [nothing per oral (NPO)] for more than a week should be considered as candidates for nutritional support. This situation may be due to a presenting medical illness or due to the type of surgery that has been done. Some patients may already be malnourished and nutritionally depleted due to either chronic starvation or an underlying disease such as malignancy, chemotherapy, or chronic debilitating medical conditions such as human immunodeficiency virus (HIV) and tuberculosis.

If any patient can tolerate enteral nourishment, then this route should be explored as the first choice. Patients should be fed orally whenever possible and as soon as possible. Patients used to be kept NPO for an extended period of time due to fear of aspiration or paralytic ileus. However, it is shown that most patients after abdominal surgery can be given oral feeds as early as 24 hours.

Certain patients may require placement of a fine bore nasogastric feeding tube, by gastrostomy or by jejunostomy. The flora in the gut is beneficial for the patient and leaves less complications and side effects compared to TPN **(Fig. 9.1)**.

If an enteral route is not possible for whatever reason, then a parenteral route is used. Initially, the peripheral vein

TABLE 9.1: Enteral nutrition solutions.

Standard	Special solutions
Ensure plus	Glucerna for diabetes
Jevity	Nepro for renal failure
Boost	Osmolite for isotonic
Promote	Vivonex for thin solution
Nutren	Crucial for critically ill
Isosource	Oxepa for sepsis, ARDS

(ARDS: acute respiratory distress syndrome)

TABLE 9.2: Parenteral nutrition.

Goals	Solutions
Volume—2,000–2,500 mL/day	Dextrose 10%, 30%, 50%
Calories—2,000–2,500 kcal/day	Amino acids 10%, 20%
Protein—100–150 g/day	Intralipid 10%, 20%, 30%
Lipids	Additives—Na, K, Ca, Mg
Electrolytes	Multivitamins, trace metals
Trace elements	
Vitamins	
Calories Calculation	
Dextrose—Volume × Percentage × 3.4. For example, 1,000 mL of D50 = 500 g = 1,700 kcal	
Lipids—Volume × Percentage × 10. For example, 500 mL of 20% intralipid = 1,000 kcal	
Amino acids—Grams of protein × 4. For example, 100 g of proteins = 400 kcal	

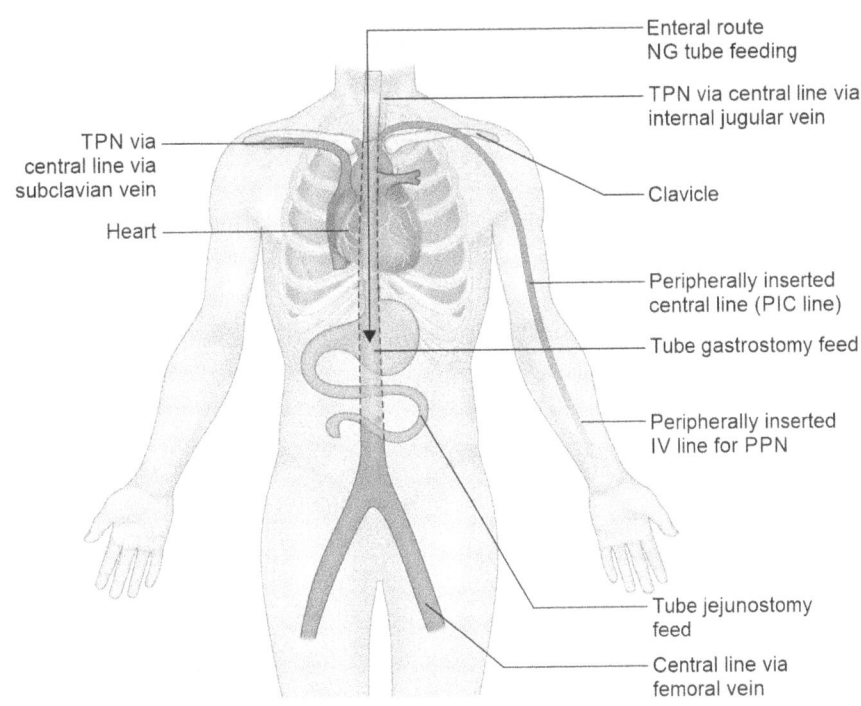

Fig. 9.1: Routes of nutritional support.
(NG: nasogastric; PIC line: peripherally inserted central catheter; IV: intravenous; PPN: peripheral parenteral nutrition; TPN: total parenteral nutrition)

can be used using less concentrated solutions. This is called PPN. However, large amounts of fluids or concentrated solutions require a central line placement. This can be done through a peripherally inserted central catheter (PICC or PIC line) or by a centrally inserted line via the jugular approach or subclavian approach (CVP line).

When ordering the TPN solution, the volume of fluid, components, calories, and additives such as trace metals, vitamins, and protein content are taken into consideration. Please see the formula of different enteral feeds and TPN solutions.

Prolonged administration of TPN can lead to various complications with metabolic problems and catheter-related problems. Hence, all patients on TPN need close monitoring, special evaluations, and ongoing adjustments. During daily rounds, the patient should be checked for intake output, fluid overload or dehydration, electrolytes, trace elements, vitamins, acid-base balance, daily weight, liver profiles, and onset of sepsis. If any issues are noted, then appropriate corrective steps are undertaken.

KEY POINTS

Do not ignore the nutritional needs of all patients. Enteral nutrition is better whenever possible. TPN is planned early on by anticipation of prolonged starvation.

CHAPTER 10

Electrolytes and Blood Gases

INTRODUCTION

Daily work in the hospital inevitably comprises evaluation of laboratory values. Every chart is checked for the most current laboratory results including the blood count, electrolytes, and blood gases. A fall in hemoglobin and hematocrit, a rise in white cell count, and changes in electrolytes, particularly potassium, and evidence of acidosis get easy attention. A lot of information on patient status and treatment changes can be decided with this information. A simple and systematic way of analyzing these results is described here.

EVALUATION OF BLOOD GASES AND ELECTROLYTES

The house physicians are the first-line healthcare providers who are bombarded with results of blood gases and electrolytes. It is a good idea to systematically analyze these results for quick interpretation and action **(Tables 10.1 to 10.4)**.

Hematocrit/hemoglobin (Hct/Hb) gives you the status of RBC count. If anemic, explore the causes and initiate corrective measures.

pH: If it is <7.3, it shows acidosis; >7.5 shows alkalosis. These can be metabolic or respiratory in origin.

Check the HCO^-/bicarbonate: If it is <25, chances are of metabolic acidosis; >28 is probably respiratory.
- Low pH with low bicarbonate is metabolic acidosis.
- High pH with high bicarbonate is metabolic alkalosis.
- Low pH with high bicarbonate is respiratory acidosis.

TABLE 10.1: Electrolyte abnormalities—sodium.

High	Low
Dehydration	Overhydration
Endocrine problems	Diabetes insipidus
Renal	Hyperglycemia
	Diuretics
Treatment	
Hydration	Hypertonic saline
Reduce sodium	Reduce fluid

Normal value: 135–145 mEq/L

TABLE 10.2: Electrolyte abnormalities—potassium.

High	Low
Acidosis	Alkalosis
Hypovolemia	Aldosteronism
Renal failure	Renal loss
Over administration	Vomiting
Adrenal hypoactivity (Addison's disease)	Diuretics
Treatment	
Calcium or HCO_3	Administer potassium
Kayexalate, Lokemia, Veltassa	Sodium chloride
Dialysis	Magnesium
Glucose and insulin	

Normal value: 4–5 mEq/L

TABLE 10.3: Electrolyte abnormalities—calcium.

High	Low
Hyperparathyroidism	Hypoparathyroidism
Alkalosis	Hyperventilation
Bone tumors	Acidosis
Cancers	Postsurgical
Vitamin overdose	
Treatment	
Hydration	Hydration
Calcitonin	Calcium administration
Diuretics	Vitamin D
Steroids	Magnesium

Normal value: 9–10 mEq/L

TABLE 10.4: Electrolyte abnormalities—magnesium.

High	Low
Renal failure	Starvation
Drugs	Hypokalemia
	Gastrointestinal loss
	Treatment
Hydration	IV magnesium
IV calcium	
Dialysis	

Normal value: 1–2 mEq/L

TABLE 10.5: Acid–base balance—acidosis.

Metabolic	Respiratory
Low pH, low HCO₃	Low pH, high HCO₃
Hypovolemia	Hypoventilation
Cardiogenic shock	Coma
Septic shock	Drug overdose
Medications	Narcotics
Diabetic ketoacidosis	Ventilatory settings
Renal failure	
Treatment	
Hydration	Antidotes for narcotics
Correct the underlying cause	Correct ventilatory settings
Judicious use of bicarbonate	Airway maintenance

TABLE 10.6: Acid–base balance—alkalosis.

Metabolic	Respiratory
High pH, high HCO₃	High pH, low HCO₃
Pyloric stenosis	Hyperventilation
Hypokalemia	Hypercalcemia
Renal causes	Hysterical
	Treatment
Hydration	Correct ventilatory settings
Metabolic support	Sedation
	Pain medications

- High pH with low bicarbonate is respiratory alkalosis.

Once you have an assessment, explore the causes of these abnormalities (**Tables 10.5 and 10.6**).

The most common causes are:
- *Metabolic acidosis:* Hypotension, hypovolemia, hemorrhage, sepsis, gangrene of bowels, diabetic ketoacidosis, and anoxia
- *Metabolic alkalosis:* Pyloric stenosis with vomiting, hypokalemia
- *Respiratory acidosis:* Inadequate ventilation, oversedation, coma
- *Respiratory alkalosis:* Hyperventilation, hypercalcemia

Once you identify the etiology, then corrective steps can be undertaken. It may be by administration of fluids, adjustment of ventilator settings, or correction of metabolic anomalies. Hold the urge to use sodium bicarbonate IV until restorative efforts are underway.

The other two things in the blood are gases: (1) pO_2 and (2) pCO_2. They give you the level of oxygen and carbon dioxide in the blood. O_2 saturation is also shown. If the O_2 saturation is low or pO_2 is low, you would look for reasons for the same—there could be inadequate amount of oxygen in the settings, airway obstruction, need for increasing the positive-end expiratory pressure (PEEP) level, or checking the chest X-ray to see if there is pneumothorax, congestion, or collapse. If so, the patients may need bronchoscopic aspiration, insertion of chest tube, etc.

If the pCO_2 is low, it indicates hyperventilation. It may need ventilator adjustments or placement of facemask.

If pCO_2 is high, it requires increase in respiratory rate by reducing sedation or adjustment of ventilator settings.

The electrolyte readings are Na, K, Cl, HCO_3^- (or CO_2), blood urea nitrogen (BUN), creatinine, and blood sugar depending on the laboratory setup.

Again, analyze the results one by one and check if any reading is abnormal. If so, find out why and what needs to be done. These may lead you to change the type of IV fluids, administer certain medications, modify IV fluid rate, necessitate consultation from other specialists, or order further tests.

KEY POINTS

Decide if it is acidosis or alkalosis, and then if this is metabolic or respiratory in origin. Find the root cause of the problem and take corrective measures. Hold off on giving bicarbonate unless needed.

CHAPTER 11

Multiple Organ Failure

INTRODUCTION

Surgical patients can end up in the intensive care units with multiple organ failures. The surgeon may be at a loss since multiple specialists are making independent decisions on patient care based on their expertise. Often, the care is delegated to the intensivist. However, the surgeon and surgical staff should be vigilant, active, and involved in care of the patient, particularly if the initial insult was related to a surgical pathology.

DISCUSSION

Surgeons are often faced with many acute surgical problems that require complex management with teamwork. Patients who have had major trauma such as an automobile accident, gunshot wounds, blast injuries, or conditions such as ruptured abdominal aortic aneurysm, major burns, acute hemorrhagic pancreatitis, massive fecal peritonitis, or severe septic shock are examples where they can become hypotensive, anuric, and go into respiratory and cardiac failure.

Multiple physicians of different specialties are likely to be involved in care of such a patient. Each physician is focused on the system of his/her expertise, and rotating junior house officers of multiple specialty may make rounds on these patients daily. If the initial pathology is a surgical condition, then it is reasonable to expect the surgical team to continue to lead the team. Very often, the management is guided by the developments during the past few hours and may be channeled toward troubleshooting those immediate problems.

If possible, all physicians, nurses, and other caregivers should make a combined round at a specified time so that a multidisciplinary discussion can be entertained about patient management. It also can be a teaching round for medical students and residents. A systematic approach to physical examination, review of the chart, and discussion with other caregivers, particularly the nursing staff, will facilitate this. Review of current and past vital signs and intake and output chart, followed by system-by-system evaluation to include cardiac, pulmonary, renal, abdominal, peripheral vascular, and neurological status is done. The most recent laboratory values are reviewed. All current medications are reviewed, and nutritional status, deep venous thrombosis (DVT) prophylaxis, decubitus care, body weight, and antibiotic coverage are evaluated.

If the patient is on a ventilator, evaluation is made as to the need for continued ventilator support, and efforts are made to see if the patient can be weaned off the ventilator.

After the rounds are completed, it may be time to take certain actions such as inserting or removing central lines, change of dressings, and other procedures such as tracheostomy, special monitoring line placements, or dialysis catheter placement; or order new tests such as chest X-ray, cultures, and special laboratory tests; or transfuse blood or blood products. Aseptic and protective precautions are observed to protect the patient as well as the caregivers. The patient may have to be moved for special studies such as computed tomography (CT) scan or interventional radiology procedures or even operating room procedures.

Immediate documentation of assessment and treatment plans are recorded on the chart, so that other caregivers may know the status. It is equally important to follow the effect of the newly instituted therapy such as a change in ventilatory settings or administering a certain drug.

Discussion with family and legal next of kin and guardians should be made at least once every day. After a period of several days in the intensive care unit, it is not uncommon for the physicians to lose sight of the big picture, being focused on the immediate settings. One should not lose hope, but at the same time, one needs to be realistic on the prognosis of individual patients.

As a rule, if there are three or more organ systems that need continued support over a prolonged period, the chance of survival is slim. One may want to initiate a conversation about a patient's living will and end of life instructions, especially if the quality of life is likely to be poor and recovery is unlikely. It will be a tremendous financial and emotional burden on the family and guardians to continue to keep someone alive with artificial life support indefinitely. Ethics committees and risk management advisers are of great help in situations of dilemma.

KEY POINTS

Surgeons should be directly involved in the continued care of the patient in the intensive care unit, if the initial pathology was surgical. Teamwork is necessary.

SECTION 2

Abdominal Pain

12. Abdominal Pain
13. Right Upper Quadrant Abdominal Pain
14. Right Lower Quadrant Abdominal Pain
15. Left Upper Quadrant Abdominal Pain
16. Left Lower Quadrant Abdominal Pain
17. Suprapubic Pain
18. Mid-Abdominal Pain
19. Severe Abdominal Pain

CHAPTER 12: Abdominal Pain

INTRODUCTION

Abdominal pain is a common presenting symptom. With a detailed history and physical examination, headway to a diagnosis can be made. Judicious and expeditious investigations can lead to the final diagnosis. Over half of the abdominal pains subside spontaneously. Only a small percentage of the remaining ones have serious or acute problems that will eventually need surgery. The abdominal viscera are supplied by the autonomic nervous system and carry no pain sensation. There are two major events that cause pain: (1) ischemia and (2) inflammation or peritonitis. Obstruction and stretching of the bowel walls cause a dull sensation and cramping that progress to ischemia or peritonitis. How to pick the real surgical cases and how to expedite their care? Sometimes, a simple physical examination is adequate to send the patient directly to the operating room. Sometimes, a few tests and radiology imaging clarify the situation.

TYPES OF ABDOMINAL PAIN

Abdominal pain is a very common symptom, and surgeons are usually asked to evaluate these patients. More than half of these patients never require any surgery. Vast majority of abdominal pains are due to medical conditions such as gastritis, gastroenteritis, acid reflux, food poisoning, viral infections and bacterial infections, parasitic infestations, menstrual cramps, pelvic inflammatory disease, endometriosis, urinary tract infections, inflammatory bowel disease, and intake of medications and alcohol. However, it is of paramount importance to examine these patients, perform necessary tests, and make sure that there are no acute surgical issues. Location of the pain, duration of the pain, and age of the patient are critical in the history **(Table 12.1)**.

Young patients often present with acute problems such as acute appendicitis, gastroenteritis, and pancreatitis. Older patients have a higher incidence of diverticulitis, malignancies, and ischemic problems.

Mid-abdominal pain can be due to gastroenteritis, food poisoning, pancreatitis, and gastric disorders. Right upper quadrant (RUQ) pain is suggestive of cholelithiasis, cholecystitis, or other liver disorders. Left upper quadrant pain is suggestive of splenic pathology or left colon ischemia. Right lower quadrant (RLQ) pain is suggestive of appendicitis or cecal lesions. Left lower quadrant pain suggests diverticulitis or colonic problems. Suprapubic pain suggests pelvic inflammatory disease or tubo-ovarian problems **(Fig. 12.1)**. Flank pain suggests renal problems or musculoskeletal problems. Back pain should raise the suspicion of abdominal aortic aneurysm (AAA) and other spinal problems. Severe abdominal pain unrelieved with pain medications should raise suspicion of a major internal catastrophe including unsuspected hernias, gangrene of bowels, volvulus, and mesenteric thrombosis. This topic is separately discussed in Chapter 19.

Tests are ordered to corroborate these diagnoses accordingly. Start with initial tests such as an ultrasound for RUQ pain to rule out gallbladder pathology, for suprapubic pain to rule out uterine and tubo-ovarian pathology, and for back pain as well as for flank pain to rule out AAA and renal problems.

TABLE 12.1: Different types of abdominal pain.

Right upper quadrant	Epigastric	Left upper quadrant
Gallbladder	Lower esophagus	Spleen
Liver	Stomach	Splenic flexure colon
Hepatic flexure colon	Peptic ulcer	
	Central	
	Pancreatitis, peritonitis, food poisoning, small bowel	
Right lower quadrant	Suprapubic	Left lower quadrant
Appendicitis	Cystitis	Diverticulitis
Cecal pathology	Endometritis	Colitis
Terminal ileum	Salpingo-oophoritis	Carcinoma

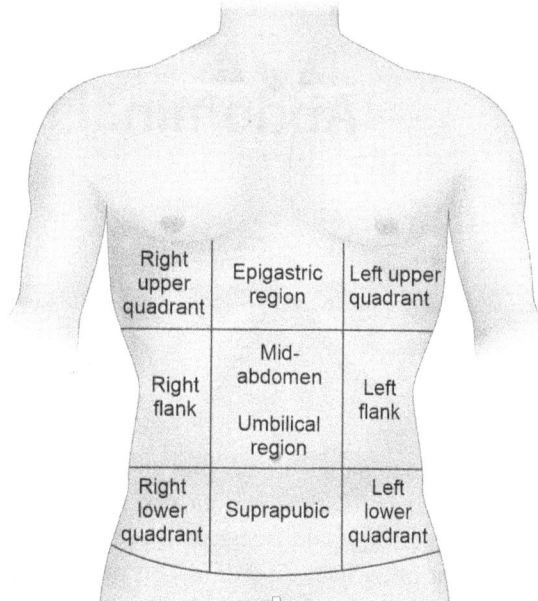

Fig. 12.1: Quadrants of abdomen.

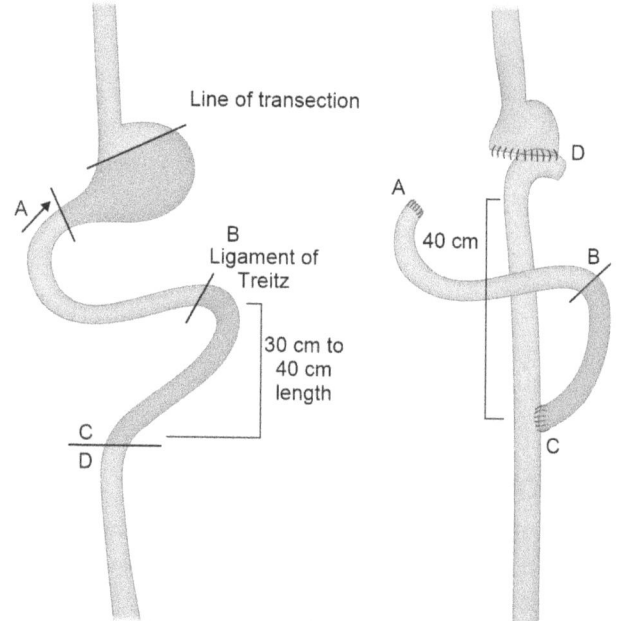

Fig. 12.3: Subtotal gastrectomy with Roux-en-Y anastomosis.

> **BOX 12.1:** Etiology and treatment of peptic ulcer.
> - *Etiology:* Helicobacter pylori, nonsteroidal anti-inflammatory agents, hydrochloric acid, bile, alcohol, smoking, stress, ischemia
> - Duodenal ulcer diathesis varies somewhat from gastric ulcer—gastric ulcer must be evaluated to ensure that there is no malignancy
> - *Medical treatment:* Antacids, sucralfate, H_2 receptor antagonists, proton-pump inhibitors, antibiotics against *H. pylori* (Amoxicillin with Clarithromycin)
> - *Surgical treatment:* Truncal vagotomy with pyloroplasty or gastrojejunostomy, highly selective vagotomy, distal gastrectomy (antrectomy) with Billroth I or Billroth II reconstruction, subtotal gastrectomy

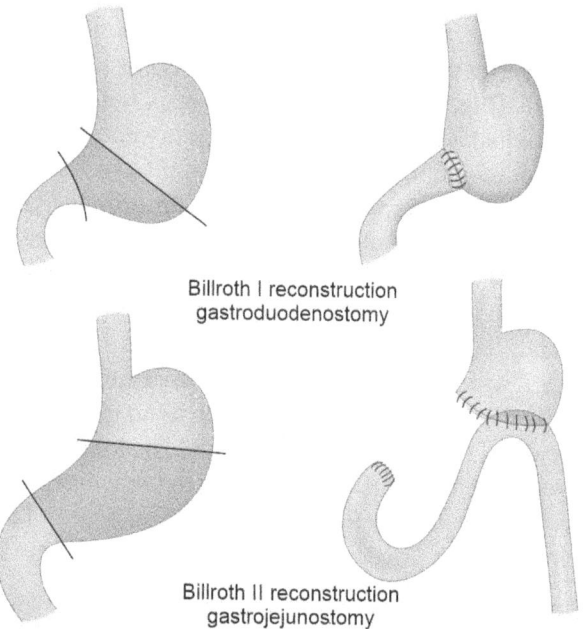

Fig. 12.2: Partial gastrectomy.

a complete measurement of electrolytes, and full chemistry panel including liver function tests, as well as amylase and lipase levels. Often, a flat and erect X-ray of the abdomen is also routinely obtained **(Figs. 12.2 and 12.3)**.

Further detailed discussion is entertained on peptic ulcer problems in **Box 12.1**.

For mid-abdominal pain, amylase and lipase tests are done to rule out pancreatitis. A computed tomography (CT) scan of the abdomen may be the best initial test for all others.

Once an idea is formed based on these tests, then additional tests are ordered as necessary, or treatment is started. All patients should get a complete blood count test,

KEY POINTS

Abdominal pain is common and resolves spontaneously in many instances. However, all patients must be fully examined and worked up to ensure that serious issues are not overlooked.

CHAPTER 13

Right Upper Quadrant Abdominal Pain

INTRODUCTION

Cholelithiasis and cholecystitis are common surgical problems; cholecystectomy is one of the common general surgical procedures performed all across the globe. The most common cause of right upper quadrant (RUQ) abdominal pain is gallbladder disorders. Symptoms can vary from vague dull upper abdominal pain with or without radiation to the back, loss of appetite, fatty food intolerance, or fever, chills, and jaundice (Charcot's triad). Chronic cholecystitis can be treated electively by doing a laparoscopic cholecystectomy. Acute cholecystitis will require hospital admission, intravenous (IV) antibiotics, and an urgent cholecystectomy. Acute ascending cholangitis is a life-threatening surgical emergency where there is bacteremia from pus in the common bile duct (CBD). Every cholecystectomy patient should be evaluated for CBD stones and associated pancreatitis before surgery.

RIGHT UPPER QUADRANT PAIN

Differential diagnosis of RUQ abdominal pain is hepatobiliary and pancreatic pathology, rarely duodenal ulcer, or right colon pathology. The most common problems are cholelithiasis and cholecystitis.

History of acute or chronic intermittent pain, fever, jaundice, and alcohol consumption is noted. A physical examination evaluates for tenderness and guarding in RUQ (Murphy's sign), palpable mass, and peritoneal signs.

A complete blood count test for hemoglobin (Hb) and white blood cells (WBC) is ordered. An elevated WBC count indicates infection. Liver function tests are ordered to note any abnormalities. Amylase and lipase tests are also requested to rule out pancreatitis **(Boxes 13.1 and 13.2)**.

The next best test to evaluate for gallbladder pathology is an ultrasound of the RUQ of the abdomen. If gallstones are present with no evidence of acute cholecystitis and the patient has no fever or tenderness, then this can be treated by elective cholecystectomy. If the patient is already admitted to the hospital and agreed for surgery, laparoscopic cholecystectomy is scheduled for the next available suitable time, such as next-day morning.

If the ultrasound examination shows evidence of acute cholecystitis, and clinical signs also corroborate with tenderness, fever, and leukocytosis, then the patient is immediately started on IV antibiotics. Emergency cholecystectomy is recommended on the same day or next day. The laparoscopic method is chosen with the understanding that there could be a higher potential for conversion to open method.

If the diagnosis is unclear, a hepatobiliary iminodiacetic acid (HIDA) scan and a computed tomography (CT) scan

> **BOX 13.1:** Cholecystitis—initial decisions.
>
> - Is it acute or chronic?—fever, leukocytosis, tenderness, sudden onset? Urgency of treatment, antibiotics, surgery
> - Are liver enzymes elevated?—may indicate common duct stones and cancers
> - Are amylase, lipase elevated?—indicates pancreatitis
> - Are there stones or not?

> **BOX 13.2:** Cholecystitis tests.
>
> - Complete blood count—Hb, Hct, WBC, platelets
> - Liver enzymes, PT, PTT, amylase, lipase
> - Sonogram—best test for stones
> - HIDA scan—best test to know if the cystic duct is obstructed or not—indicating acute cholecystitis
> - CT scan—best test for pancreas
> - MRCP—best initial test for pancreatic and bile duct
> - ERCP—both diagnostic and therapeutic for common bile duct

(CT: computed tomography; ERCP: endoscopic retrograde cholangiopancreatography; Hb: hemoglobin; Hct: hematocrit; HIDA: hepatobiliary iminodiacetic acid; MRCP: magnetic resonance cholangiopancreatography; PT: prothrombin time; PTT: partial thromboplastin time; WBC: white blood cell) are needed. Otherwise, there is no need for additional tests. The HIDA scan will show if the cystic duct is patent or not. An obstructed cystic duct can be due to a small stone or due to edema secondary to inflammation. A positive HIDA scan is one that visualizes the liver, extrahepatic biliary tree, and flow into the duodenum, but with no visualization of the gallbladder. Such a picture suggests acute cholecystitis when there is associated abdominal tenderness, fever, and leukocytosis.

If the liver chemistries are elevated, one has to decide whether this is due to a CBD stone or due to other causes of obstructive jaundice such as carcinoma of the pancreatic head, or if this is due to liver disease. A mild degree of elevation of liver chemistries can be due to the cholecystitis itself.

If the liver chemistry shows only mild elevation of liver enzymes in a patient with acute cholecystitis, one could take the patient for laparoscopic or open cholecystectomy without any additional investigations. However, a cystic duct cholangiogram will be strongly recommended at surgery to ensure that the bile duct is clean **(Fig. 13.1)**.

If the liver chemistries are significantly elevated, the next best test to do is a CT scan of the abdomen. This will rule out any lesions in the head of the pancreas and any gross pathology in the liver, CBD, and pancreas. However, it may not detect any small stones in the gallbladder or in the CBD. It may show a dilated biliary tree indicative of a blockage in the CBD. In order to further define the problem, we do an endoscopic retrograde cholangiopancreatography (ERCP) or magnetic resonance cholangiopancreatography (MRCP).

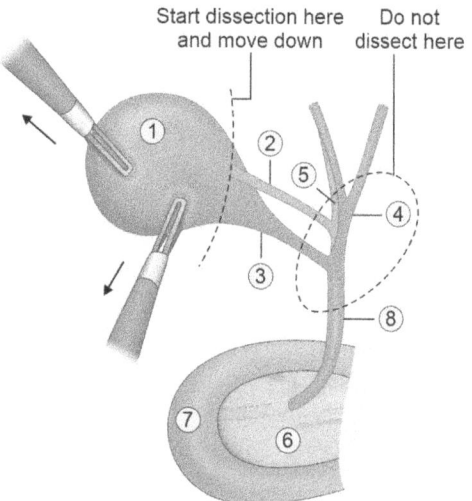

Fig. 13.1: Clear view of cystic artery and cystic duct. (1) Gallbladder, (2) cystic artery (3) cystic duct, (4) common hepatic duct, (5) hepatic artery (6) head of pancreas, (7) duodenum, and (8) common bile duct.

An ERCP can be both diagnostic and therapeutic, in the sense that one can do a papillotomy and remove CBD stones using balloon catheters or wire baskets. However, MRCP is noninvasive and can prescreen patients who really need the ERCP.

If diagnosis of CBD stones with cholelithiasis is confirmed, then one needs to plan for surgery. The choices are to either have a preoperative ERCP, papillotomy, and removal of CBD stones followed by laparoscopic cholecystectomy, or perform open cholecystectomy with CBD exploration, or for the technically comfortable surgeons to perform laparoscopic cholecystectomy and CBD exploration also done laparoscopically at the same sitting.

During cholecystectomy, if an intraoperative cholangiogram shows CBD stones, the choices are to either try and remove them at the same sitting or let the ERCP specialist remove them postoperatively. If the surgery is being done by an open method from the beginning, one should go ahead and explore the CBD, remove the stones, and close with T-tube drainage. If the surgery was by a laparoscopic method, then the CBD exploration at the same sitting depends upon the proficiency of the surgeon and availability of necessary tools. Another option is to convert the laparoscopic method to an open method and complete the procedure. This is where the surgeon has to exercise judgment based on hospital facilities, availability of tools, specialists, discussion with patient and family, and the surgeon's own comfort level.

If there are numerous CBD stones, and if complete removal and clearance of the CBD cannot be assured, one should consider doing biliary enteric anastomosis. This can be in the form of choledochoduodenostomy or Roux-en-Y choledochojejunostomy. A tightly impacted stone at the ampulla of Vater may need open transduodenal sphincteroplasty **(Box 13.3)**.

If the HIDA scan is negative, it gives more time to plan further investigation. One may do ejection fraction with cholecystokinin. This will help to identify cases of biliary dyskinesia where the ejection fraction is low.

How to treat biliary dyskinesia? One must rule out any other causes of recurrent RUQ pain and discomfort. The gastrointestinal (GI) evaluation includes upper endoscopy, and a CT scan to rule out any other hepatobiliary pathology is done. If all other tests are negative, and if the patient agrees, laparoscopic cholecystectomy is done as an elective procedure. About half of the patients feel an improvement in symptoms after the surgery.

At times, there can be evidence of acute cholecystitis without stones in the gallbladder. This could be due to acalculus cholecystitis or a small, impacted solitary stone in the cystic duct. Acalculus cholecystitis is seen on patients

> **BOX 13.3:** Treatment of cholecystitis.
>
> - *Acute:* Plan for emergency cholecystectomy, IV antibiotics, laparoscopic cholecystectomy, open procedure as standby
> - *Chronic:* Plan for elective cholecystectomy and laparoscopic cholecystectomy most of the time
> - *No stones:* If the patient is acutely ill, plan for percutaneous cholecystostomy and IV antibiotics. If the patient is not acutely ill, consider biliary dyskinesia with GI workup and consider elective laparoscopic cholecystectomy
> - *Stones present:* Plan for cholecystectomy; rule out common bile duct stones
> - *Liver chemistry elevated:* Workup to rule out common bile duct stones, cancers of bile duct or pancreas, pancreatitis, severe cholecystitis
> - *Amylase lipase elevated:* Rule out pancreatitis. Wait for pancreatitis to subside before any surgery
> - *Common bile duct stones:* Options:
>   - Preoperative ERCP papillotomy followed by laparoscopic cholecystectomy
>   - Cholecystectomy and common bile duct exploration at the same sitting by laparoscopic or open method
>   - Cholecystectomy first followed by ERCP papillotomy

(ERCP: endoscopic retrograde cholangiopancreatography; GI: gastrointestinal; IV: intravenous)

who are otherwise ill and bedridden with no oral feeds. A sonogram will be negative for stones, but will show evidence of thickened wall, and pericholecystic fluid. The HIDA scan will be positive. If the patient is acutely ill and at a poor risk for surgery, a percutaneous cholecystostomy tube can be placed under CT guidance. The patient is given antibiotics and closely monitored. An elective planned cholecystectomy can be done or at times the tube can be removed after a well-defined track has formed to the exterior.

If the CT scan shows abnormalities in the pancreas, then additional evaluations are carried out. A carcinoma of the head of the pancreas is suspected when a mass lesion is noted in this area. It can cause obstructive jaundice, elevated liver chemistry, and dyspeptic symptoms. Fine-needle aspiration (FNA) cytology of the mass can be done to confirm diagnosis. Treatment will depend upon resectability of the lesion, which would involve pancreaticoduodenectomy, also known as Whipple resection. If it is resectable, then the surgery gives the best hope. If the lesion is not resectable, then a palliative bypass such as cholecystojejunostomy, with or without a gastrojejunostomy, will reduce the jaundice and avoid gastric outlet obstruction. Chemotherapy can be added in both instances for supplemental gain.

Pancreatitis is suspected when the CT scan shows diffuse enlargement or bogginess of the pancreas. Serum amylase and lipase levels are usually elevated. Acute pancreatitis can be very severe or mild. The patient is always admitted and monitored.

If the liver chemistry shows markedly elevated liver enzymes, then one should suspect hepatitis. A specific hepatitis profile is ordered. If acute hepatitis is confirmed, a medical consultation is obtained for the best supportive measures.

Other causes of RUQ abdominal pain include inflammation or tumor of right colon, hepatic flexure or transvers colon, pathologies involving liver such as hepatitis, cirrhosis of liver, liver abscess, hepatoma, congestive heart failure, or subphrenic abscess. Investigations as described above will help in the diagnosis.

KEY POINTS

Think of gallbladder problems in RUQ abdominal pain as the first diagnosis. Look for associated pancreatitis or CBD stones. Decide if this is an emergency or can be handled electively.

CHAPTER 14

Right Lower Quadrant Abdominal Pain

INTRODUCTION

Acute appendicitis is the first consideration for patients complaining of right lower quadrant (RLQ) abdominal pain. There can be other reasons, but everyone wants to rule out appendicitis first since it is the most common condition here. The lumen of the appendix is narrow and any occlusion of the lumen due to swollen lymphatic patches, fecal ball, or worms can lead to edema, inflammation, and perforation much more easily than any other part of the gastrointestinal (GI) tract. Since it contains fecal flora with mixed organisms, this leads to peritonitis, sepsis, and abscess formation. The appendix can be in different positions in the abdominal cavity and can initially present as referred pain. In a young male patient with a typical history and localized tenderness in RLQ with rebound tenderness, one can prepare the patient for surgery of appendectomy with no other investigations. For others, one may consider doing an ultrasound examination or a computed tomography (CT) scan of the abdomen. A CT scan offers the best diagnostic imaging in confirming acute appendicitis with 95% accuracy.

PATHOLOGY AND TREATMENT

The most common pathology causing RLQ abdominal pain is acute appendicitis. Less common is inflammation of cecum due to diverticulitis of cecum, or inflammation due to parasitic infection such as amebiasis or tuberculosis. Even more rare conditions are carcinoma of the cecum or appendix, Crohn's disease of terminal ileum, and mesenteric adenitis. In female patients, one should think of tubo-ovarian pathology, and in children Meckel's diverticulitis.

A young male patient with recent onset of RLQ abdominal pain along with tenderness in this area and leukocytosis is almost certain to be having acute appendicitis. Such a patient can be directly scheduled for appendectomy without any further tests.

A CT scan of the abdomen with thin cuts is the most common diagnostic test for acute appendicitis today. If there is any question in the diagnosis, it is advisable to obtain it. In a clear clinical situation as described in the above paragraph, it is not necessary to obtain a CT scan. An alternate test is a sonogram of RLQ of the abdomen. It is less accurate than a CT scan. In many parts of the world, it is the poor man's CT scan because of cost concerns.

Once a diagnosis of acute appendicitis is made, the treatment of choice is appendectomy. It can be done by open method via a small RLQ incision or laparoscopically **(Boxes 14.1 and 14.2)**. The choice depends on the availability of necessary instruments and experience of the surgeon. In the United States, almost all cases are now done by the laparoscopic method.

During surgery, if acute appendicitis is confirmed by gross inspection, the appendix is removed with minimal contamination. It is not necessary to explore the rest of the abdomen or run the bowel to look for incidental findings.

Different methods are described and practiced in handling the base of the appendix or the appendicular

---

BOX 14.1: Acute appendicitis.

Diagnosis:
- RLQ abdominal pain, tenderness over McBurney point, low-grade fever, progressive worsening
- Elevated WBC count, sonogram helpful, CT scan is most diagnostic

Treatment:
- NPO, IV fluids, IV antibiotics. Plan for appendectomy by laparoscopic or by open method as soon as possible

Well-defined appendiceal abscess:
- CT-guided percutaneous drainage, IV antibiotics, NPO. Plan for interval appendectomy once the acute phase is over

(CT: computed tomography; IV: intravenous; NPO: nothing per oral; RLQ: right lower quadrant; WBC: white blood cell)

> **BOX 14.2:** Appendicitis—unusual situations.
>
> - *Appendix cannot be found at surgery:* Look for retrocecal appendix adherent to the back wall of cecum, previous appendectomy. Find the cecum, mobilize it completely
> - *Appendix not inflamed at surgery:* Look for other causes of pain, such as mesenteric adenitis, salpingitis, and regional ileitis. Go ahead and complete the appendectomy to avoid future problems
> - *Appendix in the hernia sac:* Appendectomy if felt safe
> - *Tumors of appendix or cecum or cecal diverticulitis:* Right hemicolectomy with primary anastomosis
> - *Necrosis of base of appendix:* Excise to healthy viable tissue of cecum and closure with staples or two-layer suture closure

stump. It does not make a difference as to how the stump is handled. It can be tied off securely, stapled, or buried with a purse string suture.

There is a school of thought to treat appendicitis with antibiotics initially and carefully follow them and to consider appendectomy only if there is no clinical improvement. This new protocol appears to be gathering momentum, allowing more planned surgery instead of rushing them to the operating room immediately upon diagnosis.

In many parts of the world, an interval appendectomy is done as an elective procedure for patients who were once suspected to have had appendicitis but it resolved spontaneously or with antibiotic therapy. The author has serious reservations on justification for doing such cases, since the appendix is noted to be appearing normal or shrunken in these cases. Either the original diagnosis was wrong or it resolved with no residual effects.

If the clinical findings show perforated appendicitis with marked tenderness, rebound tenderness, fever, and leukocytosis, the appendectomy is scheduled more urgently and the patient is given broad-spectrum antibiotics. After the appendectomy, one may drain the RLQ.

If the CT scan shows a well walled-off abscess along with a tender palpable mass in the RLQ, it is better to drain the abscess percutaneously under CT guidance first and continue the antibiotics for 1 week. Plan for an interval appendectomy after the inflammation has completely subsided or if there is lack of improvement, which may be due to the presence of a fecalith in the abscess cavity or a persistently leaking appendiceal base.

If the appendix appears to be normal and noninflamed during a surgery that was initiated for acute appendicitis, one would still go ahead and remove the appendix to avoid future diagnostic issues, and one would look for any other cause of the symptoms that mimicked appendicitis. In women, this could be a tubo-ovarian or uterine problem such as a ruptured ovarian cyst or a pelvic inflammatory disease. In young adults, one would think of mesenteric adenitis or Crohn's disease.

KEY POINTS

Acute appendicitis is the first diagnosis when a patient complains of localized RLQ abdominal pain.

CHAPTER 15

Left Upper Quadrant Abdominal Pain

INTRODUCTION

The spleen is the first thing that comes to mind when we talk about the left upper quadrant (LUQ) of the abdomen. The spleen can get enlarged to a significant size before the patient feels any pain or discomfort. This is because the enlargement is slow in progress and it can freely expand into the peritoneal cavity. There is no infection or peritonitis in most of these cases. In acute expansion of the spleen or following rupture of the spleen, there is peritoneal irritation and pain. Blood in the peritoneal cavity can act as an irritant. The left colon and splenic flexure of the colon can be a causative area when there is ischemic colitis or diverticulitis. Overall, an isolated pain of the LUQ is much less common compared to other quadrants.

SPLENOMEGALY

The spleen and splenic flexure of the colon are the two organs in the LUQ. It is less common for the patient to present with LUQ abdominal pain compared to other areas.

An enlarged spleen can often be palpated, but it is usually not tender.

Ischemic colitis can present as pain and tenderness in LUQ. These patients may also have associated bleeding per rectum.

A computed tomography (CT) scan of the abdomen would be the most logical test to obtain.

Ischemic colitis is usually self-limiting. Surgery becomes necessary only if there is evidence of perforation and peritonitis.

An enlarged spleen needs a hematological workup to find the etiology (**Box 15.1**). Many different conditions can cause an enlarged spleen. Surgery is done only upon the recommendation of a hematologist/oncologist. It is never an emergency. The splenectomy has to be planned with

> **BOX 15.1:** Splenomegaly.
>
> *Hematologic:* Idiopathic thrombocytopenic purpura, spherocytosis, hemolytic anemias, sickle cell disease, thalassemia, hypersplenism
>
> *Malignancies:* Hodgkin and non-Hodgkin lymphoma, leukemias of all types, metastatic malignancies, myelofibrosis
>
> *Other conditions:* Portal hypertension, splenic vein thrombosis, splenic cysts, splenic abscess, infectious mononucleosis, leishmaniasis, and other parasitic infestations

due caution and after splenectomy, prophylaxis against infections is recommended. Polyvalent pneumococcal vaccine is administered.

Splenic injury following trauma can present as pain in LUQ. There can also be referred pain in the left shoulder due to irritation of the left diaphragm. There may be associated fracture of left lower ribs. The splenic injury can present as a minor avulsion of the capsule, pedicle, or as transection of parenchyma. Sometimes, it can cause subcapsular hematoma, which presents as delayed rupture of the spleen. A CT scan of the abdomen is the most common diagnostic test for ruptured spleen.

In selected cases, nonoperative management with careful observation and follow-up can be done to treat injury to the spleen if the vital signs are normal and there is minimal bleeding. All others get operated in a timely manner to avoid continued blood loss and shock.

During surgery, one must completely mobilize the spleen from its bed, holding it up on its pedicle. Then a decision can be made whether to salvage the spleen by doing partial splenectomy or suturing it. Otherwise, a total splenectomy is done. When operating on a very enlarged spleen, one should ligate the splenic artery first in the lesser sac before mobilizing the spleen from its bed, to reduce blood loss. Care should be taken to avoid injury to stomach wall when ligating short gastric arteries. Mobilizing the splenocolic ligament and the splenogastric area before mobilizing the spleen from its bed will facilitate easier dissection. Use of vascular staples, hemoclips, and harmonic scalpel can reduce blood loss. Care is taken to avoid injury to tail of pancreas that can cause a pancreatic fistula. When in doubt, the splenic bed is drained with closed suction drain at the conclusion. Laparoscopic hand-assisted splenectomy and robotic-assisted splenectomy can be done with lower morbidity. The specimen is morcellated intraabdominally inside a specimen bag to remove it through a small incision.

KEY POINTS

Isolated LUQ abdominal pain is less common as compared to pain in other locations.

CHAPTER 16

Left Lower Quadrant Abdominal Pain

INTRODUCTION

The sigmoid colon is the main organ in this quadrant. The most common cause of pain in the left lower quadrant (LLQ) of the abdomen is diverticulitis. It can present in a mild, moderate, or severe form depending on the level of inflammation and associated peritonitis. Diverticula are thinned-out protrusions of the mucosa through the serosa of the bowel and can be present for years without any major symptoms. When the thinned mucosa perforates, it induces inflammation with multibacterial flora in the fecal stream. There appear to be more predilections for the disease process in Western countries compared to Eastern countries. It could be genetics, dietary habits, or bowel habits that are responsible. Besides diverticulitis, other diseases of the colon that can cause LLQ pain or discomfort include various types of colitis, ischemic disease, parasitic infestations, and carcinoma. Investigations include colonoscopy, sonogram, barium or gastrografin enema, and a computerized axial tomography (CAT) scan of the abdomen.

DIVERTICULITIS OF THE COLON

The most common condition is diverticulitis of the colon **(Box 16.1)**. The degree of diverticulitis can vary from mild pain with minimal tenderness to severe pain, severe tenderness, and peritonitis resulting in perforation. Usually, the patients are 50 years of age or older.

The history of prior episodes of pain, constipation, or fever is relevant. Other causes of pain in the left quadrant include irritable bowel syndrome, inflammatory bowel disease, parasitic infections, tubo-ovarian problems, and ureteric stones.

A physical examination will elicit the extent of tenderness, localized peritonitis, or generalized peritonitis.

A computed tomography (CT) scan of the abdomen is the most valuable immediate test. One can confirm the diagnosis and assess the extent of inflammation, formation of abscess, or perforation accurately.

> **BOX 16.1:** Diverticulitis of sigmoid colon.
>
> *Diagnosis:*
> - Left lower quadrant abdominal pain, tenderness, fever, leukocytosis. Sonogram, CT scan of the abdomen
>
> *Treatment:*
> - Mild—IV antibiotics, diet, nonsurgical management
> - Severe—IV antibiotics, one-stage resection and anastomosis after it is cooled down
> - Perforated with peritonitis—emergency surgery to resect the perforated segment, proximal colostomy, Hartmann procedure, second-stage surgery after 6 months to reconnect the bowel
> - Well walled-off abscess—CT-guided percutaneous drainage, followed by surgical resection after it is cooled off, possible primary anastomosis, or anastomosis with proximal ileostomy
>
> (CT: computed tomography; IV: intravenous)

A complete blood count to look for leukocytosis and basic chemistry is obtained.

Treatment depends on the severity of diverticulitis. All patients are started on broad-spectrum antibiotics, since the colonic flora is multibacterial. One must cover Bacteroides, gram positives, and gram negatives.

Mild diverticulitis often subsides completely with a course of antibiotics. The patients can be followed clinically. The patient with severe diverticulitis without perforation or abscess is treated with antibiotics first and then taken up for surgery, if there is no complete resolution. With proper bowel preparation, the patients can often be treated with one-stage resection and anastomosis after resecting the infected segment. Laparoscopic hand-assisted and robotic-assisted colon resections are becoming popular.

Perforated diverticulitis with peritonitis will need emergency surgery. In these cases, resection of the perforated segment with proximal end colostomy and closure of distal stump as Hartmann's closure is the best option. After a period of 4–6 months, the bowel continuity can be re-established.

A well walled-off abscess is first drained percutaneously under CT guidance and broad-spectrum antibiotics are

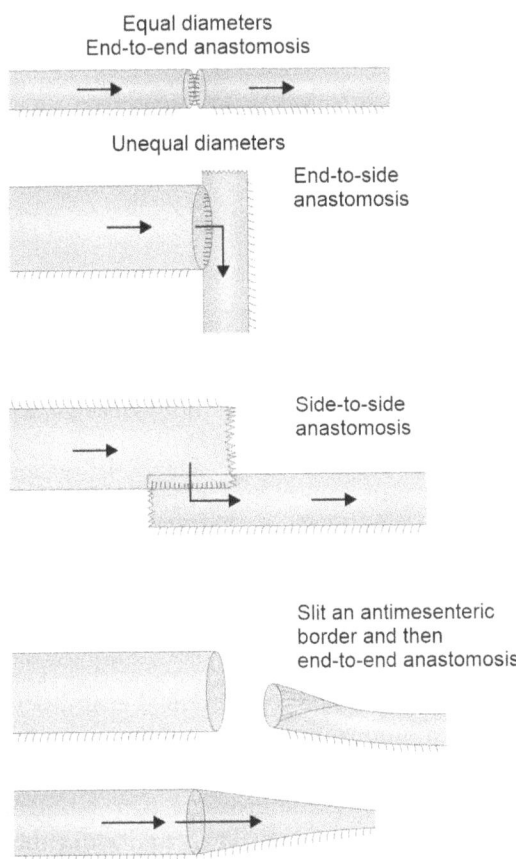

Fig. 16.1: Bowel anastomosis.

BOX 16.2: Colon resection.

- For benign conditions, one can stay close to the colonic wall and resect only the necessary segment and do primary anastomosis at any level
- However, for malignant conditions, one has to resect lymph nodes and fat and go down to the base of the arterial supply, necessitating resections along superior mesenteric or inferior mesenteric arterial distribution
- *Preconditions for anastomosis:* The cut edges should have good vascularity, no disease at cut ends (cancer, infection, granuloma), ends should come together easily with no tension and it should be technically sound watertight closure
- Proximal diversion (colostomy or ileostomy) when the anastomosis is tenuous or under emergency situations or when primary anastomosis is not done
- Diameter disparity can be overcome by doing end-to-side anastomosis or side-to-side anastomosis or by fish mouthing the narrow end along the antimesenteric side to make it an end-to-end anastomosis

given. After the inflammation has subsided, with proper bowel preparation, a one-stage resection and anastomosis can be attempted **(Fig. 16.1** and **Box 16.2).**

KEY POINTS

Acute diverticulitis is the most common problem when someone complains of LLQ abdominal pain.

CHAPTER 17

Suprapubic Pain

INTRODUCTION

Women are more prone to getting suprapubic pain. Obviously, the female organs of the pelvis are the major factor. Sometimes, it is just menstrual cramps. Sometimes, it is a ruptured ovarian follicle during ovulation resulting in bleeding into the pelvis, known as Mittelschmerz. It can also be endometriosis or salpingo-oophoritis. Other times, it could be severe pelvic inflammatory disease (PID) with endometritis. The vast majority of these patients need only antibiotic therapy. For diagnostic confirmation, sonogram and laparoscopy are done. Urinary problems with cystitis of different types are the next common reason for pelvic pain. A burning pain on micturition and a urinalysis showing white blood cells (WBC) and bacteria are useful hints in diagnosis.

PELVIC INFLAMMATORY DISEASE

The organs in the pelvic area are the urinary bladder, uterus, ovaries, and fallopian tubes. On rare occasions, an appendicitis presenting to the midline area or a sigmoid diverticulitis flapping to the midline can also present as pain in this area.

The most common problem, however, is tubo-ovarian uterine pathology such as PID in women. Sexually transmitted diseases, particularly *Chlamydia* infection, are considered in the etiology. They can subsequently lead to narrowing of the fallopian tubes, leading to infertility or ectopic pregnancy.

After history-taking and a physical examination, one would order an ultrasound of the pelvis almost routinely. Pelvic and cervical tenderness along with elevated WBC count and low-grade fever are corroborative of the diagnosis of PID. They are usually treated with antibiotics—Vibramycin® (doxycycline) together with cephalosporins. If there is any doubt in diagnosis, a diagnostic laparoscopic examination is done.

Infections of the urinary bladder can be multifactorial. A urinalysis will show bacteria and WBCs. A urine culture is confirmatory. The initial treatment is with antibiotics and then look for sources of cystitis.

KEY POINTS

Think of PID or bladder problems when a patient complains of suprapubic pain. An ultrasound would be the first-line investigation.

CHAPTER 18: Mid-Abdominal Pain

INTRODUCTION

Many patients complain of mid-abdominal pain, vague crampiness, indigestion, dyspepsia, and nausea. A majority of these symptoms are nonspecific and self-resolving. These could be due to food poisoning, acute gastritis, food allergies, alcohol intake, aspirin, or nonsteroidal analgesics. But one must keep in mind more serious conditions such as acute pancreatitis or bowel obstructions. Many other inflammatory processes start out as central or periumbilical pain and then localize to the area of actual infection. Every patient needs to be fully evaluated before discharge with antacids or analgesics.

MID-ABDOMINAL PAIN

Mid-abdominal pain is the most common type of abdominal pain. Fortunately, the vast majority of them is nonspecific in nature. The cause could vary from indigestion, gastritis, gastroenteritis, food poisoning, small bowel colic, or adhesions with partial obstruction. It is important to rule out acute pancreatitis. One must obtain serum amylase and lipase levels in all abdominal pain cases. This is the only way to make the diagnosis of pancreatitis.

If the physical examination does not show any evidence of peritonitis, then a computed tomography (CT) scan would be in order. This single test gives the maximum information. A routine flat and upright X-ray of the abdomen will give valuable information about bowel obstruction, free air, and status of the small and large bowels.

The severity of pancreatitis can be assessed from the CT scan. In addition, hematocrit (Hct), base deficit, and serum calcium levels along with pulse rate, blood pressure, and urine output are used as criteria.

The treatment in acute pancreatitis has been "to put the pancreas at rest" by keeping the patient nothing per oral (NPO) and administering intravenous (IV) fluids for fluid replacement. Close monitoring is established. Pancreatitis is a chemical burn of the retroperitoneum and not an infectious condition. Hence, there is no requirement to give IV antibiotics for the management of acute pancreatitis unless there is evidence of superadded infection by parameters such as fever, leukocytosis, bacteremia, or abscess formation. A severe necrotic pancreas may require debridement of the necrotic tissue after it has matured **(Box 18.1)**.

The investigation should also look for gallstones or CBD stones. Liver chemistry and an ultrasound of the gallbladder may be ordered. If there is evidence of gallstone pancreatitis, then a laparoscopic cholecystectomy is done after the pancreatitis has subsided.

Small bowel obstructions need admission and observation. A nasogastric (NG) tube is inserted, IV fluids are administered, and a follow-up X-ray is ordered every 24 hours. Today, the most common cause of small bowel obstruction is intra-abdominal adhesions from prior surgery. Many of the partial bowel obstructions resolve with bowel

---

BOX 18.1: Diagnosis and treatment of acute pancreatitis.

Diagnosis:
- Mid-abdominal pain, radiation to back, mild tenderness with no peritonitis, dehydration. Elevated serum amylase and lipase. CT scan of abdomen is highly diagnostic. Sonogram to rule out gallstones

Treatment:
- NPO, IV fluids, monitoring vital signs, and laboratory results. Watch Hb, Hct, calcium, oliguria, TPN, or postpyloric enteral nutrition. No need for antibiotics
- *Gallstone pancreatitis:* Elective laparoscopic cholecystectomy after pancreatitis has cooled off

(CT: computed tomography; Hb: hemoglobin; Hct: hematocrit; IV: intravenous; NPO: nothing per oral; TPN: total parenteral nutrition)

rest and decompression. If they do not resolve in 2 or 3 days, or if they are severe, surgery is needed. If the patient did not have any prior surgery, then one should look for hernias or cancers as the cause.

KEY POINTS

Most mid-abdominal pain is self-limiting and simple. Do not miss acute pancreatitis—do serum amylase and lipase tests for all abdominal pains.

CHAPTER 19

Severe Abdominal Pain

INTRODUCTION

Excruciating abdominal pain should not be treated with morphine or other analgesics. Such narcotic analgesics can mask the signs and symptoms for a close follow-up and may cause serious problems that require emergency surgery. Patient consent taken under the effect of sedatives will also be questioned later.

Major diagnostic criteria to consider are perforated viscus, peritonitis, internal hernia, volvulus with gangrene of the bowel, superior mesenteric artery occlusion with gangrene of the small bowel, midgut volvulus from malrotation, and acute hemorrhagic pancreatitis. Medical conditions of acute porphyria and abdominal crisis of autoimmune or parasitic infections are held in differential diagnosis.

PERITONITIS

When a patient is complaining of excruciating abdominal pain that is unrelieved by pain medications, one must be alert. Serious intra-abdominal problems could be present.

Peritonitis secondary to perforation of the bowel such as perforated peptic ulcer, perforated appendicitis, perforated diverticulitis, midgut volvulus with gangrene of the small bowel, internal herniation with ischemic bowel, mesenteric ischemia with gangrene, intussusceptions with ischemia, torsion of the ovary, torsion of appendix epiploicum, perforated gallbladder, ruptured liver abscesses, and ruptured tumors are all the possibilities **(Box 19.1)**. There is associated evidence of free fluid, blood, bile, bowel contents, stool, or air in the peritoneal cavity.

Examination will show the patient to be in severe distress along with signs of sweating, cold and clammy skin, tachycardia, hypotension, and oliguria. The abdomen will be tense and tender with rigidity or guarding. Rebound tenderness and absence of bowel sounds will be noted.

A plain X-ray of the abdomen showing a gasless bowel pattern is ominous. It could indicate that all the loops are filled with fluid, with no transmission of air. On the other hand, it may show free air in the abdominal cavity, indicative of a perforated bowel.

BOX 19.1: Peritonitis—acute abdomen pain.

- These are conditions that cause diffuse abdominal pain, generalized tenderness, diffuse guarding and rigidity, absent bowel sounds, fever, leukocytosis, tachycardia, and dehydration. CT scan is the test of best value
- Patients need emergency laparotomy except in cases of acute hemorrhagic pancreatitis. The causes include perforated peptic ulcer, perforated appendicitis, perforated diverticulitis, gangrene of small bowel, perforated cecum, perforated sigmoid colon or rectum, perforated small bowel, anastomotic leaks, internal hernia with strangulation, ruptured gallbladder, ruptured liver abscess, ruptured distal esophagus, torsion of ovarian cyst, mesenteric artery occlusion, ruptured liver or spleen, ruptured urinary bladder, and primary peritonitis

(CT: computed tomography)

These patients can go into septic shock quickly. A computed tomography (CT) scan of the abdomen can provide valuable information. An ultrasound can evaluate the pelvic organs or identify free fluid.

Preparation must be made for emergency laparotomy, whether a diagnosis is reached or not. Severe and excruciating abdominal pain unrelieved by narcotics must be explored. Broad-spectrum antibiotics and fluid replacement are started.

During surgery, a careful exploration is made to identify the pathology and corrective steps are undertaken. This may be to suture the perforation, resect the involved part, drain the abscess, or divert the bowel as directed during surgery.

Occlusions of the superior mesenteric artery result in gangrene of the small bowel and right half of colon, following the distribution of that artery. Very proximal one foot of jejunum will be vascularized through collaterals from the celiac axis. This condition has over 90% mortality.

> **BOX 19.2:** Gangrene of bowel.
>
> - Totally dead bowel must be resected, except in a very elderly person having total gangrene of small bowel and right colon resulting from occlusion of the superior mesenteric artery
> - Segmental gangrene caused by internal herniation, tight adhesion, or volvulus can be safely resected and reanastomosed
> - Gangrene caused by superior mesenteric artery occlusion is a result of late diagnosis. Efforts can be made to do embolectomy or bypass procedures, or infusion of papaverine and heparin if diagnosed before full-blown necrosis of the bowel wall. Usually, proximal one foot of jejunum and left colon are spared and in younger patients efforts can be made to support short gut syndrome with TPN and eventual hope for intestinal transplant
> - Patchy gangrene in segments is due to low flow syndrome from shock and poor perfusion with use of vasopressors. Second-look procedures are justified for eventual resection of necrotic tissues

(TPN: total parenteral nutrition)

All necrotic and devitalized bowels must be resected for survival, but this results in short bowel syndrome which requires massive administration of fluids, electrolyte management, and nutritional support. Gangrene of the bowel from adhesion, internal hernia, and volvulus can be easily resected and primary anastomosis performed **(Box 19.2)**.

Torsion of an ovarian cyst may require a salpingo-oophorectomy. Perforated gallbladder and perforated appendix are removed.

One of the complications of surgery for severe intra-abdominal catastrophe is development of the abdominal compartment syndrome in the postoperative period. Often, the bowels are distended; there is third spacing of fluid and swelling of all soft tissues. The abdomen may have been closed tightly. The patient develops hypotension and oliguria despite correction of the presenting pathology. A high index of suspicion must be maintained. Pressure in the urinary bladder can be measured and pressure of 30 cm of water or more is diagnostic of the abdominal compartment syndrome. The best treatment is to open the abdominal cavity, let all the bowels bulge out, and cover it with a membrane, with either plastic or biodegradable sheets, and place wound vacs or multiple drains in the peritoneal cavity, to evacuate the tissue fluid. After a period of 3 weeks, the abdominal wall can be closed by secondary closure.

KEY POINTS

Do not ignore severe abdominal pain. It is not normal. Consider immediate investigations and plan for possible surgery.

SECTION 3

Abdominal Conditions

20. Mass in the Abdomen
21. Abdominal Distension
22. Abnormal Air
23. Back Pain
24. Flank Pain
25. Jaundice
26. Anemia
27. Vomiting
28. Diarrhea
29. Heartburn: Acid Reflux
30. Obesity
31. Hematemesis

CHAPTER 20

Mass in the Abdomen

INTRODUCTION

Complete examination of each and every patient must be done irrespective of the presenting complaints. This should include palpation of the abdomen for any masses, enlarged liver, or spleen. Abdominal masses are more often discovered by the doctor rather than the patient. Any mass other than an enlarged liver or spleen should raise suspicion of possible advanced cancers. A careful assessment of the features of the mass such as its size, location, mobility, pulsation, reducibility, and associated lymphadenopathy is done to get a clinical impression. This can be further confirmed with an ultrasound examination or a computed tomography (CT) scan of the abdomen.

ABDOMINAL MASSES

Whenever we feel a mass in the abdomen, the first thing that comes to mind is cancer **(Box 20.1)**. It is an important diagnosis to be ruled out by definitive evaluations. Other possibilities include an intussusception or fecal material in a thin person. A mass in the right upper quadrant (RUQ) could be a palpable enlarged liver or an enlarged gallbladder. A mass in left upper quadrant (LUQ) could be an enlarged spleen. A mass in right lower quadrant (RLQ) could be related to the appendix or cecum. A mass in the mid-abdomen could be related to the pancreas or stomach **(Box 20.2)**.

Intussusception in children can present with a mass in the RLQ. A mass in the left lower quadrant (LLQ) could be a tumor of the sigmoid colon or sometimes it is just fecal mass in the colon.

A mass in the suprapubic region can be a distended urinary bladder or an enlarged uterus related to either pregnancy or a tumor.

A pulsatile mass in the epigastric region could be related to an abdominal aortic aneurysm (AAA). However, it can also be a palpable aorta on a thin person. The differentiation is made by evaluating whether it is expansile impulse or transmitted pulsation.

Ideally, intra-abdominal gastrointestinal (GI) malignancy should be diagnosed in early stages when they are non-palpable, to hope for curative resection. Once they become palpable, they are generally advanced malignancies.

In all these cases, the best test that yields maximum information is a CT scan of the abdomen. However, routine blood tests and ultrasound examinations are often done as the first step. Additional investigations such as endoscopy or CT-guided biopsies are ordered later if required. Depending on the final diagnosis, appropriate surgery is planned.

A carcinoma of the stomach, colon, or rectum is ideally resected for cure. If curative resection is not possible, then palliative resection or bypass procedures are done. Lymph nodular masses, as in advanced lymphomas, are best treated with chemotherapy and radiation. Retroperitoneal tumors

BOX 20.1: Mass in the abdomen.
- Right upper quadrant—liver, gallbladder
- Epigastric—stomach, aortic aneurysm
- Left upper quadrant—spleen, left colon
- Mid-abdomen—pancreas
- Right lower quadrant—cecal, ileocecal, appendiceal
- Suprapubic—urinary bladder, uterus, pregnancy
- Left lower quadrant—sigmoid colon, cancers, stool

BOX 20.2: Hepatomegaly.
- Hepatitis viral
- Metabolic disorders
- Hematological disorders
- Congestive heart failure
- Cirrhosis liver
- Autoimmune disorders
- Genetic disorders
- Parasitic infections—amebiasis, malaria, hydatid cyst
- Nonparasitic liver infections and abscess
- Primary liver tumors
- Metastatic liver disease, carcinoma of gallbladder

may need a combination of radical surgery with radiation and chemotherapy.

Sometimes masses are due to benign conditions. An abscess can be well walled off resulting from acute appendicitis or acute diverticulitis. They can be evaluated with a sonogram or CT scan. If confirmed, a CT-guided needle aspiration and percutaneous drainage using a pigtail catheter can be done along with antibiotic therapy. Once the abscess is resolved, interval surgery to remove the appendix or perforated segment of colon can be done.

Pseudocysts of the pancreas can evolve as a sequel of acute pancreatitis. This is a loculated collection of ascitic fluid or peripancreatic fluid without an epithelial lining. This is opposed to true cysts of the pancreas. Pseudocysts can be initially observed for possible spontaneous resolution. If they remain persistent and become well walled, drainage can be done internally or externally.

KEY POINTS

A mass anywhere in the body needs an evaluation and investigation. The best tests are a sonogram and a CT scan. Consider doing fine-needle aspiration (FNA) cytology if it is safe. Do not aspirate or do FNA, if you suspect aneurysms or pheochromocytoma.

CHAPTER 21: Abdominal Distension

INTRODUCTION

For many patients, the initial presenting symptom is a bloating sensation of the abdomen. This can be nonspecific related to multiple conditions, or it may be the initial symptom of bowel obstruction. Fat, fluid, feces, fetus, and flatus are the classic five causes. Recent-onset distension associated with abdominal pain should be evaluated for surgical pathology. Slow progressing chronic distension will need a full metabolic workup. Treatment depends on the etiology and urgency of the clinical condition. Obesity and pregnancy should be easier to recognize.

ETIOLOGY

Fluid refers to ascites. This can be due to portal hypertension, cirrhosis of the liver, underlying alcohol addiction, end-stage liver disease for any reason, Budd–Chiari syndrome, metastatic malignancy, pancreatic pathology, or malnutrition. Fluctuation and shifting dullness can be palpated in a clinical examination. Confirmation is by a sonogram or computed tomography (CT) scan. A needle aspiration or paracentesis can be done to obtain a sample of the fluid to perform cytology and chemical analysis (Box 21.1).

Flatus refers to intestinal obstruction. Usually, there is associated abdominal pain, constipation, and emesis. Dilated loops of the small bowel or colon may be palpable or show visible peristalsis in a thin abdomen.

The etiology could be a bowel obstruction from adhesions related to a previous surgery, internal or external herniation, cancer of the colon, volvulus, or intussusception. Megacolon and toxic megacolon can be obstructive or nonobstructive. In the pediatric population, Hirschsprung's disease and imperforated anus or atresia of the gastrointestinal (GI) tract needs to be kept in mind. Senile patients and comatose patients may not know about the long-standing constipation (Box 21.2).

EVALUATION

When evaluating bowel obstruction, one has to differentiate between mechanical obstruction, paralytic ileus, and nonobstructive colonic distension. The bowel sounds are classically absent in paralytic ileus and there is an associated history of recent abdominal surgery or systemic shock.

> **BOX 21.1:** Ascites.
> - Free fluid in the peritoneal cavity, large enough to cause abdominal distension
> - Evaluate for portal hypertension, cirrhosis liver, alcohol addiction, metastatic malignancy, tuberculosis, and pancreatic pathology
> - *Tests:* Liver chemistry, coagulation profile, complete blood count, CT scan of abdomen, paracentesis with fluid sent for cytology and chemistry
> - *Treatment:* Treat underlying cause, repeat abdominal paracentesis, peritoneojugular shunt procedure

(CT: computed tomography)

> **BOX 21.2:** Intestinal obstruction.
> - Small bowel obstruction versus colonic obstruction
> - Mechanical obstruction versus paralytic ileus versus pseudoobstruction (nonobstructive megacolon)
> - *Causes:* Adhesions from prior surgery, hernia internal or external, malignancies, volvulus, intussusception, inflammatory processes, gallstone ileus, intraluminal objects, strictures, fecal impaction
> - *Tests:* Blood counts and full chemistry, X-ray of abdomen flat and upright, gastrografin enema, colonoscopy, CT scan of the abdomen
> - *Treatment:* IV fluids, NG tube decompression. Prepare for surgery, corrective surgery as needed. Urgent surgery if peritonitis is noted, if hernia internal or external is suspected, or if ischemia of bowel is suspected. IV Reglan for paralytic ileus. Colonoscopic decompression for nonobstructive megacolon

(CT: computed tomography; IV: intravenous; NG: nasogastric)

One can give intravenous (IV) Reglan (metoclopramide) and continue nasogastric (NG) tube decompression until bowel sounds return.

In the nonobstructive megacolon, there is evidence of generalized distension of the entire colon with stool noted in the sigmoid or rectum. Enema, manual evacuation of the stool, and rectal tube decompression may help. Sometimes, colonoscopic decompression is recommended, especially when the cecum is nearing 10 cm in diameter. At this level of distension, there is a chance for the cecum to rupture. After the colonoscopic decompression, a long intraluminal rectal tube can be placed for continued decompression.

A plain X-ray of the abdomen will show the dilated small bowel loops with air-fluid levels and a stepladder pattern of gas shadows, or dilated colon as the case may be. Other tests of importance are gastrografin enema, sigmoidoscopy, or colonoscopy. A follow-up CT scan of the abdomen will confirm the obstruction and level of obstruction with proximal dilated loops, distal collapsed loops, and area of transition or causative factor.

In mechanical small bowel obstruction, the bowel sounds are more prominent with visible peristalsis, as the bowels are trying to overcome the obstruction. Bowel obstruction that is persistent needs surgical correction before it becomes an emergency, such as perforation or ischemia. The exact nature of surgery depends upon the operative findings **(Box 21.3)**.

> **BOX 21.3:** Adhesions in abdomen.
>
> - Simple adhesions can be taken down; however, dense adhesions of chronic and nonobstructive nature are best left alone
> - *Technique:* To do lysis of adhesions expose both proximal and distal parts of the bowel first, start with easy spots first, inspect both front and back sides of adhesion, use sharp and blunt techniques, use traction and countertraction, do gentle handling, avoid injury to bowel as best as possible, irrigate locally, go a little bit at a time until it is completely done
> - *Prevention:* Topical instillation of different pharmacological agents and bioabsorbable membrane has been tried. Best prevention is gentle handling, good surgical techniques, good hemostasis, laparoscopic methods, absorbable sutures, irrigation of abdomen, avoid infections and spillage, avoid foreign body, preservation of peritoneum and omentum as much as possible, avoiding unnecessary dissections, and expeditious procedure

KEY POINTS

Abdominal distension needs careful evaluation. The main thing to address immediately would be bowel obstructions. Ascites is a medical problem, most commonly related to cirrhosis of the liver.

CHAPTER 22

Abnormal Air

INTRODUCTION

Normally, air is present in the respiratory tract and gastrointestinal (GI) tract. A small amount of air is present in the paranasal sinuses and the middle ear. If air appears in any other part of body tissues, it would be abnormal. Sometimes, it is innocuous and self-resolving, but sometimes it is serious and a sign of a life-threatening state. Air in the subcutaneous tissue can be felt as eggshell crackling crepitus on palpation. Air in the bowel wall is noted on X-rays. Air in the biliary tree can be a sign of sepsis or biliary enteric communication. Air in the peritoneal cavity could be postsurgical or a sign of a perforated viscus. Air in the portal vein is a terminal sign of pylephlebitis. Air in soft tissues can be seen in gas gangrene, abscesses, and necrotizing infections. It is important for the surgeon to evaluate any abnormal air and decide on the next course of action.

AIR IN THE BODY

Air in the Peritoneal Cavity

Free air in the peritoneal cavity usually means perforations of hollow viscus. It could be in the lower end of the esophagus, stomach, duodenum, small intestine, or large intestine including the upper rectum. Following abdominal surgery, either by open or by laparoscopic method, free air can remain trapped in the peritoneal cavity for a period of 1 week. If the patient had no history of recent abdominal surgery and there is a complaint of severe abdominal pain, presence of free air is an adequate indication to perform an exploratory laparotomy. If there is no abdominal pain or tenderness and the patient looks completely comfortable with normal vital signs, one may do a computed tomography (CT) scan or gastrografin study of the stomach for further evaluation. Once in a while, a very high lying hepatic flexure or splenic flexure abutting against the diaphragm can give an erroneous appearance of free air. Another possibility is that a microperforation appeared and got sealed off immediately by the omentum.

At surgery, a careful search is made to identify the site of perforation. The presence of bile-stained fluid with GI contents points to a duodenal or gastric ulcer perforation. A duodenal ulcer perforation can be repaired with an omental patch for reinforcement (Roscoe–Graham patch). A gastric ulcer can be malignant and needs either resection or biopsy with appropriate reconstruction. The small bowel can have diverticula or pneumatosis intestinalis. The cecum can get perforated due to distal obstruction, toxic megacolon, or volvulus. It is best to do a right hemicolectomy with primary anastomosis between terminal ileum and transverse colon. A perforated appendicitis does not give rise to free air in the abdomen. A perforated sigmoid colon is usually due to acute diverticulitis. These would require resection, with proximal colostomy and closure of the distal end as Hartmann's closure. After a period of 4–6 months, a second-stage repair can be done to restore bowel continuity. Perforation of rectum or left colon can occur during colonoscopy or sigmoidoscopy. These can be primarily repaired since they usually have a good bowel cleansing already and they are detected soon after the injury.

Once in a while, it may not be easy to find the area of perforation. Typhoid perforation of the small bowel can be very tiny. One should look at the back wall of the stomach by opening the lesser sac. Insertion of a nasogastric (NG) tube and instilling methylene blue into the stomach can help to find the area of leak. Distal esophageal perforation is rare and can be repaired primarily if there is no malignancy. Check the mesenteric edge of the small and large bowel closely since small perforations can be hiding in the mesenteric fat.

Air in the Gallbladder and Common Bile Duct

The main concern would be severe infection with gas-forming organisms. Emphysematous cholecystitis occurs when the gallbladder is distended and thick walled, sometimes showing air in the wall of the gallbladder, along with an air-fluid level inside the gallbladder. These patients need emergency cholecystectomy since gangrene of the gallbladder with perforation is impending. Air can be seen in the biliary tree when there is acute ascending cholangitis where there is pus inside the common bile duct (CBD), usually associated with stones in the CBD. These patients need immediate hydration, broad-spectrum intravenous (IV) antibiotics, and removal of CBD stones with drainage of the bile duct, either by endoscopic retrograde cholangiopancreatography (ERCP) and papillotomy with stent placement or by open surgery. Biliary enteric communication can give rise to air inside the bile duct. This can happen following cholecystoduodenal fistula or after a surgical biliary enteric anastomosis, such as choledochoduodenostomy or cholecystojejunostomy.

Air in the Mesenteric Vein, Portal Vein and Inside Liver

This is an ominous sign of impending mortality in many cases. It is indicative of gangrene of the bowel or extreme bacteremia. The patient will need broad-spectrum IV antibiotics, systemic support, and evaluation for life-saving measures. Emergency laparotomy is a consideration.

Air in Soft Tissues

Gas bubbles in the soft tissue can be seen in the X-ray in cases of severe necrotizing fasciitis, gas gangrene, and diabetic necrotizing abscesses. These are caused by gas-forming organisms. Emergency wide radical debridement of the infected areas along with IV antibiotic coverage is needed. It may be necessary to do amputations at a healthy level to save the life of the patient. A large dose of penicillin along with coverage against gram-negatives will be needed. Systemic support against septic shock is required.

Surgical Emphysema

Surgical emphysema is the term used to describe air that has seeped into the subcutaneous tissues. It feels as if crackling soap bubbles or eggshells, with a special feel of crepitus on palpation. It is commonly seen following laparoscopic procedures, especially after prolonged procedures or when the gas leaks into preperitoneal space. This will dissolve spontaneously after 1 or 2 days. It is more serious following chest trauma, when there is puncture of the lung and fracture of the rib, with air from the lung injury seeping into the subcutaneous space often associated with pneumothorax. The pneumothorax is treated with placement of a chest tube. The surgical emphysema will dissolve by itself after a period of several days. Air bubbles may be seen in the mediastinum following injury to the esophagus or pharynx, following instrumentations, stab wounds, gunshot wounds, or spontaneous rupture of the esophagus (Boerhaave's syndrome). Drainage of the mediastinum, surgical repair of the wound, and antibiotic therapy are recommended.

KEY POINTS

Air is abnormal when seen in the peritoneal cavity, soft tissues, mediastinum, veins, biliary tree, or subcutaneous areas. They must be investigated and treated.

CHAPTER 23

Back Pain

INTRODUCTION

Almost everyone gets back pain sometime or other in his or her life. Fortunately, most of them are due to muscle sprain from lifting or strenuous activity and they resolve spontaneously. However, it is important to recognize more serious problems such as a herniated disc, fractured vertebrae, metastatic cancers, or ruptured aneurysms and take early action in treating them.

BACK PAIN

Back pain is a very common problem affecting a large population. The main task is to differentiate musculoskeletal problems from a herniated disc. A history of recent heavy lifting or strenuous activity combined with relief upon rest and aggravation with movement or certain postures would suggest muscular pain. Most back pain requires only nonsurgical treatments consisting of pain medications, physiotherapy, and back exercises. Such cases will resolve spontaneously. Obesity, postural habits, lack of regular exercise, sleeping habits, and psychological problems are contributing factors for back pain.

From an orthopedic/neurosurgical point of view, one would like to rule out prolapsed intervertebral disc with impingement on nerve roots. They would order a magnetic resonance imaging (MRI) of the spine. If the pain does not resolve with rest, physiotherapy, and pain medications, or if neurological deficits such as muscle weakness occur, then they will need surgery. Focused decompression of the nerve root canal by doing discectomy is adequate.

Fractures of the vertebra following falls or trauma need immediate immobilization and neurological evaluation for spinal cord injury. The patient may go into neurogenic shock and need intravenous (IV) fluids to maintain blood pressure. Shock could also be due to associated injuries and internal damage. Use of steroids is controversial but recommended to reduce neurological edema. Plain X-rays, a computed tomography (CT) scan, and MRI are useful tests. Strict immobilization is maintained until the patient can be transferred to a spine specialist or a neurosurgeon. Those with unstable spinal injuries will need operative fixation.

Infections in the spinal or paraspinal regions can also cause back pain. There may be history of prior surgery to the spine resulting in osteomyelitis, history of systemic sepsis, or tuberculosis with cold abscess. An MRI of the spine would be useful. Antibiotic therapy along with drainage of the septic focus is needed.

Metastasis to the spine is a possible phenomenon. The spread is via the bloodstream. History of cancers such as breast, prostate, lung, and thyroid is elicited. X-rays may show lytic lesions in many of them. Prostate cancer metastasis shows as denser spots. Treatment is directed to the primary cancer and radiation or chemotherapy. Certain malignancies such as multiple myeloma can present as osteolytic spots in the spine with back pain. Retroperitoneal sarcomas or lymphomas can also present as back pain.

Osteoporosis leads to loss of the bone matrix resulting in compression fractures and back pain. It could be due to lack of adequate calcium intake, vitamin deficiencies, hyperparathyroidism, hyperthyroidism, hormone changes of low estrogen or testosterone, short bowel syndrome, or medications. They need correction of nutritional deficiencies and calcium supplementation. Osteoarthritis and spinal stenosis from aging are held in differential diagnosis. Back pain can also occur as a result of spinal abnormalities such as kyphosis or scoliosis.

From a vascular surgeon's point of view, one would like to rule out a ruptured abdominal aortic aneurysm (AAA). The patient experiences sudden excruciating and nonrelenting back pain unrelieved by pain medications and is associated with sweating, tachycardia, and hypotension. Getting an immediate CT scan of the abdomen or a bedside ultrasound examination of the abdomen makes a confirmation.

KEY POINTS

Most back pains are simple problems. However, do not miss a ruptured AAA in an acute setting.

CHAPTER 24

Flank Pain

INTRODUCTION

Flank pain is felt more toward the lumbar region of the back, below the rib margin. It can be on one side alone or bilateral. Renal pathology is the most common reason for flank pain. Acute infections such as pyelonephritis come as the first diagnosis. Physical examination shows tenderness over the renal angle. Other causes can be paraspinal infections, tuberculosis, musculoskeletal sprains, lumbar hernias, or retroperitoneal tumors. Urinalysis, blood tests, sonogram, and a computed tomography (CT) scan are the most useful diagnostic measures.

FLANK PAIN

Flank pain is different from back pain. Back pain is felt in the center of the back over the spine and paraspinal regions. Flank pain is felt more to the side of the back, near the lumbar region.

The organ located here is the kidney. The most common reason for flank pain would be pyelonephritis. There can be several causes of urinary infection such as kidney stones, reflux from bladder, pregnancy induced, or indwelling Foley catheter.

Urinary tract infections are more common in women. Causes of cystitis include sexually transmitted infections, pregnancy, urethritis, calculus disease, diabetes mellitus, neurogenic bladder, nonspecific etiology, and prostatitis in men. They complain of burning pain on micturition, frequency, hesitancy, and urgency. The urine could have a foul odor. The patient may have associated fever or chills.

Culture of urine and microscopic examination of the urine may show bacteria. Sonogram of the kidneys will show stones, hydronephrosis, or other abnormalities of the urinary collecting system. Blood culture may show bacteremia.

The common types of kidney stones are comprised of calcium, uric acid, struvite, or cysteine. They present with acute colicky pain or dull flank pain that waxes and wanes. Radiation of the pain can go down to the pelvis, back, or abdomen. Associated symptoms of nausea, vomiting, hematuria, and fever are possible. Initial medical therapy includes adequate pain control, hydration, dietary advice, and antibiotics if there is associated infection. For those with obstructing stones, treatment modalities include shock wave lithotripsy (SWL), percutaneous nephrolithotomy (PCNL), endoscopic retrieval, and open surgery. Nephrectomy may be needed for those who have a loss of renal function with pyonephrosis.

Treatment is with intravenous (IV) antibiotics, usually requiring broad-spectrum coverage. The underlying etiology that caused the infection needs to be addressed. A urology consultation is requested for any interventions.

Tumors of the kidney must be ruled out in all cases. A sonogram followed by a CT scan should confirm the diagnosis. Tumors of the kidney would require radical nephrectomy.

Rare causes of flank pain include lumbar hernia, shingles, nerve root compression, and fracture of the vertebrae.

KEY POINTS

Renal angle tenderness usually indicates urinary tract infection.

CHAPTER 25

Jaundice

INTRODUCTION

Jaundice refers to a yellowish discoloration of the sclera, skin, urine, and mucous membrane due to increased levels of bilirubin. This can be due to an increased load of bilirubin from heme breakdown called prehepatic jaundice, disease of the liver called hepatic jaundice, or inability of bile to flow out caused by obstruction of the bile duct called posthepatic jaundice. The bilirubin can be conjugated and called direct bilirubin which happens in obstructive jaundice, or it can be unconjugated and called indirect bilirubin which happens in prehepatic jaundice. Jaundice is a sign of how the liver and biliary system work. It needs workup, investigations, and treatment. It could be a simple self-resolving condition such as neonatal jaundice or a complex and life-threatening condition such as cancer of the head of the pancreas.

TABLE 25.1: Jaundice—etiology.

Prehepatic	Hepatic	Posthepatic
Increased bilirubin load	Liver disease	Obstructed bile duct
Hemolytic anemia	Cirrhosis	Stones in bile duct
Newborn jaundice	Hepatitis	Cancer of pancreas
Spherocytosis	Toxins	Cancer of bile duct
Gilbert syndrome	TPN	Sclerosing cholangitis hemobilia
Blood transfusions	Drugs	Mirizzi syndrome
Crigler–Najjar syndrome	Storage disorders	Liver cancers
		Metastatic cancers
		Intrabiliary parasites

(TPN: total parenteral nutrition)

CASE AND MANAGEMENT

The patient says, "I am turning yellow."

Bile is yellow. The patient turns yellow when the bilirubin level in the blood goes up. This could be because of an increased production of bile pigments in the blood due to hemolytic anemia (prehepatic), or if the liver is not able to function well due to diseases of the liver (hepatic or intrahepatic), or if the bile is not able to flow out of the liver as in obstruction of the bile duct (posthepatic or obstructive jaundice). The surgeon is most commonly confronted with posthepatic or obstructive jaundice **(Table 25.1)**.

A history of recent onset of painless jaundice along with a palpable gallbladder in the right upper quadrant of the abdomen (Courvoisier's gallbladder) should point toward an obstructed common bile duct (CBD). The stool is clay colored in obstructive jaundice.

Liver function tests will show a high level of bilirubin and how much of it is direct and indirect (conjugated or unconjugated), along with levels of alkaline phosphatase and transaminases [serum glutamic-oxaloacetic transaminase (SGOT) test, serum glutamic-pyruvic transaminase (SGPT) test] **(Box 25.1)**. A high level of conjugated or direct bilirubin with elevated alkaline phosphatase and normal or mildly elevated transaminases point to obstructive pathology. High levels of transaminases and indirect bilirubin point toward a hepatitis-type disease.

The next test will be an ultrasound of the gallbladder to know if there are stones in the gallbladder or CBD and to know if the gallbladder or CBD is dilated or not. The presence of stones in the gallbladder or stones in the bile duct points to calculus disease.

A computed tomography (CT) scan is done next to rule out pancreatic tumors involving the head of the pancreas **(Box 25.2)**. Carcinoma of the head of the pancreas must be ruled out. It is also the best test to assess resectability of the pancreatic tumor if present.

Magnetic resonance cholangiopancreatography (MRCP) is often done at this point to evaluate the bile

56 SECTION 3: Abdominal Conditions

> **BOX 25.1:** Jaundice—blood tests.
> - Bilirubin level—conjugated (direct) high in obstructive jaundice, nonconjugated (indirect) high in others
> - Transaminase enzymes very high in hepatitis. Mildly elevated in others
> - Alkaline phosphatase elevated moderately in obstructive jaundice. Mildly elevated in others
> - Proteins (albumin) decreased in liver diseases
> - Prothrombin time elevated in liver diseases
> - Red cell count decreased in liver diseases
> - Hepatitis serum assay—confirmatory for different types of hepatitis

> **BOX 25.2:** Jaundice—investigations.
> - Ultrasound—good for gallstones, CBD stones, gallbladder wall, and pericholecystic fluid
> - CT scan—good for all abdominal viscera, liver, head and body of pancreas, metastatic disease, fluid in the abdomen
> - MRCP—good for entire biliary tree, pancreatic duct, gallbladder, portal area
> - Transhepatic cholangiogram—excellent for visualization of biliary tree from liver down
> - Intraoperative cholangiogram—excellent for visualization of bile duct and assuring patency during surgery
> - ERCP—valuable in both diagnostic and therapeutic abilities. Visualizes duodenum, ampulla, bile duct, and pancreatic duct. Can do papillotomy, stent placement, remove CBD stones

(CBD: common bile duct; CT: computed tomography; ERCP: endoscopic retrograde cholangiopancreatography; MRCP: magnetic resonance cholangiopancreatography)

duct and pancreatic duct in a more focused way and to decide on a more invasive test of endoscopic retrograde cholangiopancreatography (ERCP). ERCP can be diagnostic and therapeutic in certain situations. Papillotomy of the biliary ampulla and removal of CBD stones can be done, or a stent can be placed in the bile duct to drain the bile as the case may be.

Once all of the tests are completed, surgery is planned based on the exact diagnosis. If there are stones in the CBD, cholecystectomy and removal of the CBD stones are done. This can be done by open surgery or by laparoscopic method depending upon various factors **(Boxes 25.3 and 25.4)**. If there are numerous stones in the bile duct and they cannot be removed to full satisfaction, then a biliary enteric anastomosis can be done, such as choledochoduodenostomy or Roux-en-Y choledochojejunostomy **(Boxes 25.5 and 25.6)**.

> **BOX 25.3:** Jaundice—treatment.
> - Find the underlying cause and treat accordingly
> - All patients need nutritional support, correction of coagulation abnormalities, avoid hepatotoxicity in choosing medications, correction of anemia, and stop alcohol use
> - Surgical interventions for obstructive pathology, depending on nature and site
> - All others are treated medically. Consider use of immunoglobulins. Effective antiviral medications for hepatitis C includes Sovaldi, Harvoni, and Olysio
> - Very high bilirubin is life-threatening, with hepatorenal syndrome and multisystem failure. Liver transplantation and extracorporeal perfusion in dire situations

> **BOX 25.4:** Common bile duct stones—treatment.
> - *Preoperative ERCP* and papillotomy, removal of CBD stones, possible stent placement, followed by cholecystectomy by open or laparoscopic method with intraoperative cholangiogram
> - Open or laparoscopic cholecystectomy and common bile duct exploration at the same sitting with T-tube drainage of CBD
> - *Postoperative ERCP* for retrieval of residual or leftover stones in CBD
> - Biliary-enteric anastomosis, either choledochoduodenostomy or Roux-en-Y choledochojejunostomy for multiple numerous recurrent stones in CBD, Caroli's disease
> - Duodenotomy, sphincteroplasty for stones tightly impacted at the ampulla

(CBD: common bile duct; ERCP: endoscopic retrograde cholangiopancreatography)

> **BOX 25.5:** Carcinoma of head of pancreas—diagnosis.
> - Painless obstructive jaundice of short duration, weight loss, loss of appetite
> - Palpable gallbladder (Courvoisier's gallbladder)
> - Elevated direct bilirubin, alkaline phosphatase
> - Sonogram showing dilated gallbladder and bile duct
> - CT scan showing tumor head of pancreas
> - MRCP showing similar findings
> - ERCP showing inability to cannulate bile duct or pancreatic duct
> - Fine aspiration cytology under CT guidance

(CT: computed tomography; ERCP: endoscopic retrograde cholangiopancreatography; MRCP: magnetic resonance cholangiopancreatography)

If it is found to be secondary to a tumor of the pancreatic head or a tumor of the distal bile duct, then a radical resection is done, which would involve a Whipple resection **(Fig. 25.1; Box 25.7)**. Otherwise, a palliative bypass procedure such as cholecystojejunostomy is done.

If the diagnosis is medical jaundice such as hepatitis or cirrhosis of the liver, a medical consultation is obtained

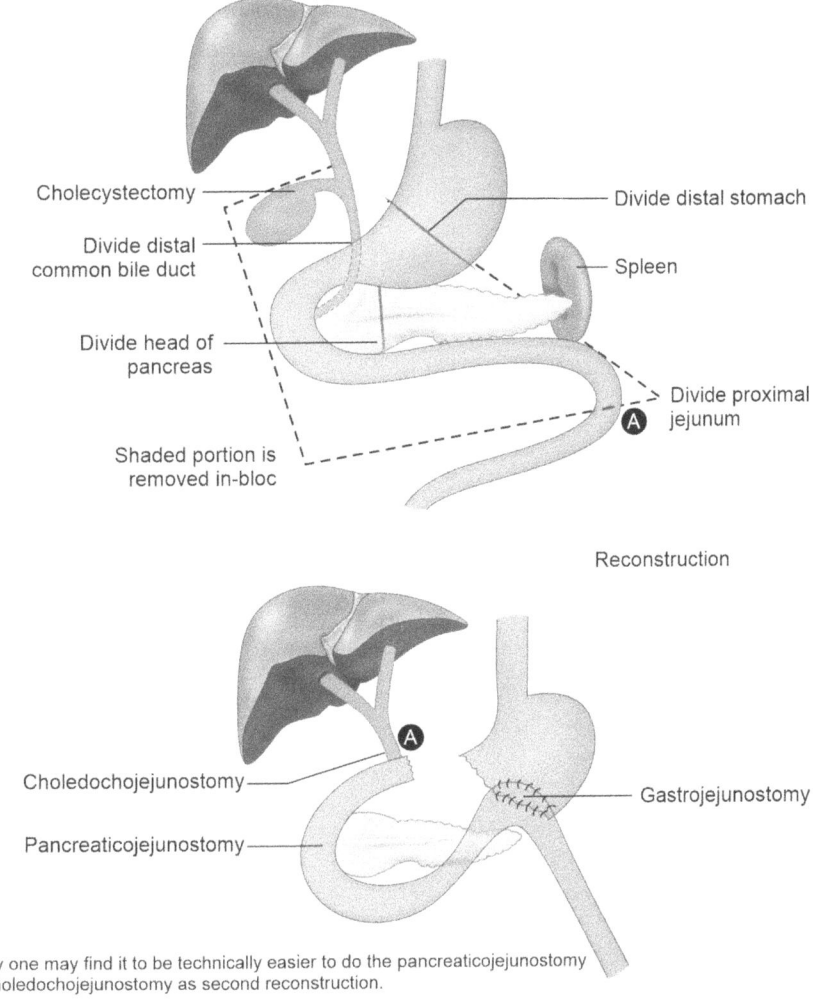

Fig. 25.1: Whipple resection—pancreaticoduodenectomy.

BOX 25.6: Carcinoma of head of pancreas—treatment.

Assess operability and resectability of the tumor. Take into consideration age and general condition of the patient, as well as patient's and family's wishes.
CT scan with thin cuts is the best test for preoperative evaluation:
- Look for any evidence of metastasis
- Evaluate size and extent of tumor
- Look at the space behind the head of pancreas toward vena cava
- Look at the space between the uncinate process and superior mesenteric artery and vein. The tumor should be resectable for cure and should be free of superior mesenteric artery and vein, portal vein, and vena cava

Curative resection by radical pancreaticoduodenectomy (Whipple resection) offers the best chance for cure
If curative resection is not possible, plan for *palliative procedures* such as biliary enteric bypass or biliary stent placements

(CT: computed tomography)

BOX 25.7: Whipple resection.

- *Indication:* Carcinoma of head of pancreas, carcinoma of distal common bile duct, periampullary carcinoma, carcinoma of duodenum, severe trauma to head of pancreas with bleeding
- *Contraindication:* Metastatic disease, invasion or dense adhesion of tumor on to portal vein, vena cava, SMA/SMV, poor general condition
- *Technique:* Mobilize duodenum after Kocher maneuver, assess resectability and relationship to superior mesenteric vessels and vena cava, clear lesser curvature of stomach, do cholecystectomy, clear dissect the distal common bile duct, mobilize ligament of Treitz and separate third and fourth parts of duodenum up to the superior mesenteric vessels, transect distal stomach, transect distal common bile duct, transect first part of jejunum at ligament of Treitz, separate head of pancreas from superior mesenteric vein and artery, ligate and divide gastroduodenal artery and create the passageway under neck of pancreas overlying portal vein, transect neck of pancreas at this line, bring the fourth part of jejunum under the SMA/SMV toward right side, separate the uncinate process, and remove the specimen. Reconstruction is by pancreaticojejunostomy, choledochojejunostomy, and gastrojejunostomy

(SMA: superior mesenteric artery; SMV: superior mesenteric vein)

for supportive care. Most of these require nutritional care, correction of metabolic abnormalities, and antiviral treatments as the case may dictate.

KEY POINTS

Jaundice could be due to medical problems such as cirrhosis of the liver, hepatitis, an obstructed CBD secondary to CBD stones, cancer of the head of the pancreas, or cancer of the bile duct. Liver chemistry and a CT scan of the abdomen followed by MRCP or ERCP should help in diagnosis and probable therapy. Surgery is carefully planned for final treatment.

CHAPTER 26: Anemia

INTRODUCTION

Anemia is low red blood cell (RBC) count. It could be due to sudden acute blood loss or slow and chronic blood loss. Anemia must be investigated and treated. The causative factor could be medical conditions, but it could also be due to surgically treatable problems. Many colorectal cancers and ulcerative conditions of the gastrointestinal (GI) tract start out as anemia. The patient looks pale, has shortness of breath, and feels weak. The urge to treat the patients by giving a blood transfusion should be curtailed unless there is ongoing rapid blood loss.

EVALUATION AND MANAGEMENT

A low RBC count is confirmed by a simple blood test. The patient looks pale and conjunctiva is pale.

The main effort is to diagnose the cause of blood loss. A hemoccult test will show evidence of slow GI tract bleeding. This may be from a peptic ulcer, cancer in the stomach, or a colorectal tumor. If hemoccult is positive, one must follow it up with an upper and lower GI endoscopy **(Table 26.1)**.

In women, one should look for excessive menstrual bleeding which could lead to more important gynecological pathology.

It is possible that the anemia is due to medical problems such as nutritional deficiencies, bone marrow disorders, neoplasia, or hemolytic anemia. One may suggest getting a hematology consultation in these cases. Some of these patients with conditions such as hereditary spherocytosis, myelodysplasia, thrombocytopenia, and selected cases of neoplasia may be benefited by splenectomy.

More often, one observes anemia in patients admitted in the hospital with major medical and surgical problems. Following trauma, major surgery, or blood loss situations, it takes several days for the body to equilibrate.

Major sepsis, prolonged hospitalization, chemotherapy, renal failure, and frequent blood draws in the hospital are factors that can contribute to anemia.

Some of these patients need a blood transfusion; however, judicious use of transfusion is recommended **(Box 26.1)**. Hemoglobin < 7 is usually held as a critical level for transfusion. It is well proven that patients who receive transfusions are at a higher risk for a variety of complications and higher mortality. Hence, anemia is best treated with medications and correction of the underlying reason for anemia. This may involve nutritional support and the use of

TABLE 26.1: Anemia—etiology.

Blood loss	Hemolytic	Aplastic
Cancers of GI tract	Neonatal	Bone marrow depression
Peptic ulcer	Spherocytosis	Myelodysplasia
Menorrhagia	Mismatch transfusion	Leukemia
Trauma	Drug reaction	Chemotherapy
Ruptured aneurysm	Autoimmune	Immune suppression
Ectopic pregnancy	Allergic	Metastatic disease
Acute pancreatitis	Sickle cell disease	Drug reaction
Renal failure		
Nutritional		
Severe illness		

BOX 26.1: Anemia—tests and treatment.

- Peripheral smear, complete blood count, liver profile
- Bone marrow aspiration
- GI workup—upper and lower endoscopy
- Identify the cause of anemia and correct same
- Stop the bleeding
- Iron (enteral and parenteral), erythropoietin, vitamins, folic acid, dietary changes
- Transfusion when Hb is <7
- Use of blood substitutes

(GI: gastrointestinal; Hb: hemoglobin)

enteral or parenteral iron, erythropoietin, vitamins, and rare elements.

In situations of acute blood loss such as ruptured aortic aneurysm or trauma, one should not wait for the hematocrit or hemoglobin results. Blood loss that is obvious should be replaced with blood as soon as possible. It will take 48 hours for the body to equilibrate hemoglobin and hematocrit. In these situations, transfusion of whole blood is preferable. If components are being used, replacement at a 1:1:1 ratio of packed RBCs, plasma, and platelets is recommended.

At times, one may come across a patient who refuses blood transfusion due to religious or personal beliefs, despite severe anemia and need for major surgery. Efforts are made to correct anemia using bone marrow stimulants, medications, nutritional support, and iron and vitamins. Minimally invasive procedures are chosen if possible. Autotransfusion of own blood is set up when blood loss is expected. Blood substitutes and artificial blood are used when the need arises.

KEY POINTS

Find the cause of anemia before starting a transfusion. Hold the transfusion unless hemoglobin is < 7 or if it is affecting vital signs. Correct the underlying cause and treat medically as far as possible. Many patients tolerate chronic anemia and low hemoglobin well.

CHAPTER 27: Vomiting

INTRODUCTION

Emesis is a common symptom associated with multiple problems and generally classified as either central nervous system in origin or abdominal in origin. It can be anything from food poisoning to bowel obstruction, alcoholism to brain tumor. A careful history and physical examination with judicious investigations will define etiology that is often associated with nausea. Treatment can also be in two categories: (1) those directed at the gastrointestinal (GI) tract and (2) those directed to the central nervous system.

ETIOLOGY AND DIAGNOSIS

Emesis is a sign of revolt by the GI tract in response to an insult to the body. One can divide this into two main categories: (1) caused by a systemic problem or (2) caused by a local pathology.

Systemic problems can be conditions such as a migraine headache, intracranial lesions, head injuries, uremia, drug toxicity or drug reactions, vertigo, labyrinthitis, postanesthetic recovery, chemotherapy medicines, and stressful or fearful emotions **(Table 27.1)**.

TABLE 27.1: Causes of emesis.

Central causes	Local causes
Postanesthesia	Acute gastritis
Head trauma	Acute gastric dilatation
Migraine	Intestinal obstruction
Labyrinthitis	Pyloric stenosis
Uremia	Pregnancy
Stress and fear	Intra-abdominal infections
Intracranial tumors	Peritonitis
Vertigo	Jaundice and liver problems
Chemotherapy	Bulimia
Drug toxicity	Drugs, poisons
Hyperemesis gravidarum	Food poisoning

Local conditions are bowel obstructions, pyloric stenosis, acute gastritis, acute gastric dilatation, poisonings, alcohol intake, jaundice, pregnancy, and any acute intra-abdominal pathology or inflammations.

Intestinal obstruction is a major concern for the surgeon when the patient presents with vomiting. It can be due to intraluminal blockage caused by gallstone (gallstone ileus), malignancies, tuberculosis, parasitic infections, food bolus, or bezoars. It can be due to bowel wall pathology such as Crohn's disease, ulcerative colitis, tuberculosis, malignancy, or ischemia. It can also be extramural pathology such as hernia, adhesive bands, volvulus, intussusception, or extrinsic compressions.

A careful history and physical examination can lead to suspicious causes. Nausea is an associated symptom. Investigations such as a plain X-ray of the abdomen, blood tests, and a computed tomography (CT) scan will show more evidence. A specific examination to evaluate the stomach itself would be an upper GI endoscopy. Certain specific conditions such as hyperemesis gravidarum, bulimia, and nonspecific hyperemesis need to be kept in mind when other conditions are ruled out.

Projectile vomiting in the newborn children can be due to congenital hypertrophic pyloric stenosis. The pyloric sphincter is very thick and acts as an obstructive valve. Usually, symptoms start a few days after birth, typically characterized by sharp projectile vomiting after feeding milk. A thickened olive size mass can be palpated in the right upper quadrant. Diagnosis can be confirmed by gastrografin study. Treatment is by surgical pyloromyotomy, taking care to avoid perforation of the mucosa. The prognosis is generally good.

TREATMENT

Treatment is directed to the underlying cause and corrective steps **(Box 27.1)**.

> **BOX 27.1:** Emesis—treatment.
>
> - Nasogastric tube to decompress the bowel and to prevent aspiration
> - Find the etiology and correct the same—surgery if needed
> - IV fluids, electrolyte monitoring
> - Antiemetic medications—Zofran, Phenergan, Vistaril, Compazine
> - Nutritional support—TPN or postpyloric feeding

(IV: intravenous; TPN: total parenteral nutrition)

A nasogastric tube is inserted to decompress the bowel and to prevent aspiration. Intravenous (IV) fluids are given to maintain the fluid balance, and electrolyte balance is monitored.

Hypokalemic, hypochloremic metabolic alkalosis is noted following emesis related to pyloric stenosis. It needs replacement of chlorides and potassium along with IV fluids.

Nutritional needs are to be addressed in the form of total parenteral nutrition (TPN) or partial parenteral nutrition (PPN). Certain patients may be in a catabolic state with chronic malnutrition. Whenever possible, enteric alimentation and vitamin supplements are addressed.

Surgical interventions may be needed if a correctable pathology is identified. Pyloric stenosis is treated with partial gastrectomy or gastroenterostomy. Releasing the obstructions such as lysis of adhesions or release of hernia corrects small bowel obstructions. Sometimes, appropriate bowel resections or bypass procedures are done. Sometimes, surgery such as feeding gastrostomy or jejunostomy is performed to maintain nutrition.

Meanwhile, symptomatic control is attempted with the use of antiemetics such as Zofran®, Phenergan®, Emetrol®, or Compazine®. These antiemetic medications are especially useful during postanesthetic care and those with central nervous system causes of emesis. Patients receiving chemotherapy need regular antiemetic medications. Those with metastatic malignancies need hospice care and sedations.

Nutritional support needs attention in protracted emesis, in the form of TPN.

KEY POINTS

Decide if the vomiting is due to a systemic problem or due to GI problems. Antiemetics are good for immediate relief, particularly for emesis of central nervous system origin.

CHAPTER 28

Diarrhea

INTRODUCTION

Frequent liquid bowel movements can be disabling and cause dehydration, electrolyte imbalance, and renal failure. It could be sudden in onset such as acute food poisoning, acute gastroenteritis, or dysentery. It can be chronic and constant in situations such as Crohn's disease, ulcerative colitis, or short bowel syndrome. Certain situations such as *Clostridium difficile* (*C. difficile*) are nosocomial infections created by abuse of antibiotics. A careful history and physical examination along with study of the stool and blood can assist in diagnosis.

ETIOLOGY AND MANAGEMENT

Loose bowel movements are abnormal symptoms of absorptive function of the gastrointestinal (GI) tract, which can be due to either excretion of excessive fluid into lumen or decreased reabsorption of expected fluid.

Drugs that have a laxative effect cause excessive fluid to be secreted into the lumen of intestines. Enteral alimentation with higher osmolality or volume can be responsible. Short bowel syndrome, resection of terminal ileum, or subtotal colectomy can cause reduced reabsorption of water or bile salts from the colon.

Medical conditions such as cholera, human immunodeficiency virus (HIV), food poisoning, and a variety of other infectious conditions cause irritation of the intestinal mucosa.

Diarrhea with excessive excretion of fat is steatorrhea, which can be the result of pancreatic problems or immune disorders. Stool can be analyzed for fat content, as well as for ova or parasites.

Inflammatory bowel diseases such as Crohn's disease or ulcerative colitis need to be ruled out in long-standing diarrhea in young patients.

Clostridium difficile is a suspect for inpatients who received antibiotic therapy. Analysis of the stool specifically for *C. difficile* titer is diagnostic. Endoscopy shows hyperemia, edema, redness, and pseudomembranous whitish patches, also called pseudomembranous colitis.

Underlying pathology needs to be corrected to effectively treat the symptoms of diarrhea. This may require antibiotics for infectious conditions such as Salmonellosis or stoppage of antibiotics in *C. difficile* patients. Specific medications directed at the problem may be needed, such as vancomycin or Flagyl® for *C. difficile* patients (**Box 28.1**).

Crohn's disease and ulcerative colitis are initially treated with medications such as Azulfidine® or Remicade® along with careful surveillance. Many of them may require eventual surgery such as subtotal colectomy or bowel resections.

Clostridium difficile diarrhea can at times progress to toxic megacolon, systemic sepsis, perforation, peritonitis, and death (**Box 28.2**). These patients need to be monitored carefully in isolation care and critical care settings with multisystem support. A daily X-ray of the abdomen is taken to look for free air in the abdomen or air in the wall of the colon, as well as to measure the diameter of cecum. Surgical intervention will be necessary before it progresses to a critical state. The best surgery is subtotal colectomy with ileostomy and closure of rectal stump. More recently, ileostomy with colonic lavage has been tried.

Intravenous fluids to replace loss of body fluid are important in conditions such as cholera. Loss of absorptive

> **BOX 28.1:** Diarrhea—treatment.
> - Find the cause and treat the underlying disease
> - IV fluids, electrolyte monitoring
> - Antibiotics for infectious diarrhea and *Clostridium difficile*—Vancomycin, Flagyl, Cipro, fidaxomicin
> - Medications—Questran, Sulfa meds, Kaopectate, Lomotil, Bismuth kaolin, Imodium
> - Isolation, hand washing, prevention of cross contamination
> - Surgical correction for inflammatory bowel disease

(IV: intravenous)

> **BOX 28.2:** *Clostridium difficile* colitis.
>
> - It is *caused by* sporeforming, grampositive, anaerobic bacteria occurring as a nosocomial infection related to antibiotic abuse due to suppression of normal bacterial flora in the colon
> - It produces *toxin A and B*, which causes pseudomembranous colitis resulting in severe diarrhea, toxic megacolon, perforation, peritonitis, and death if untreated
> - *Diagnosis:* Stool for *Clostridium difficile* titer, flexible sigmoidoscopy
> - *Treatment:* Oral Metronidazole (Flagyl), oral Vancomycin, Fidaxomicin, IV immunoglobulin, probiotics, stop other antibiotics, isolation, handwashing and efforts to reduce stool contamination, fecal transplant, NPO, and TPN
> - *For toxic megacolon surgery:* Subtotal colectomy with ileostomy, loop ileostomy with colonic lavage with polyethylene glycol

(IV: intravenous; NPO: nothing per oral; TPN: total parenteral nutrition)

> **BOX 28.3:** Causes and treatment of constipation.
>
> - *Causes:* Elderly, demented, medications, habitual, dietary, intestinal obstruction, carcinoma of colon, congenital megacolon, acquired megacolon, fecal impaction
> - *Treatment:* Treat underlying causes, disimpaction of stool, laxatives, enemas, barium enema, evacuation studies, colonoscopy
> - Surgery for malignancies, megacolon to include colectomy or colostomy

function following resection of the terminal ileum will require Questran® to bind the bile salts. Isolation of patients, prevention of cross contamination, and hand washing are emphasized in the hospital **(Box 28.3)**.

Last but not least are symptomatic medications to firm the stool. Common prescriptions are Kaopectate® (bismuth subsalicylate), Lomotil®, or Imodium®.

KEY POINTS

Decide on the etiology of diarrhea. Short duration is usually due to infectious diseases. Chronic ones are due to inflammatory bowel diseases or other GI pathologies. Cross contamination precautions, nutritional support, and intravenous (IV) fluid replacements are to be considered. Short-term help with medications is often prescribed.

CHAPTER 29

Heartburn: Acid Reflux

INTRODUCTION

Many patients refer to heartburn as acidity in the epigastrium or chest. True enough, there is acid reflux from the stomach to lower esophagus. There is associated hiatal hernia to account for this. The lower esophageal sphincter is patulous and it is in the chest cavity rather than below the diaphragm. The condition is also referred to as gastroesophageal reflux disease (GERD).

HEARTBURN

Heartburn is usually due to esophagitis, gastritis, or hiatal hernia. Regurgitation of food is a common symptom. Acid refluxes into the lower esophagus cause irritation of the mucosa and eventually cause inflammation, stricture, and metaplasia. This causes persistent heartburn symptoms, regurgitation, sleep apnea, and eventual aspiration.

Alcohol intake, excessive use of nonsteroidal anti-inflammatory agents, and certain types of food such as tomato paste, fatty food, or spicy food can aggravate the condition.

TESTS

- Gastrografin swallowing studies to demonstrate reflux and hiatal hernia
- Upper endoscopy to evaluate for esophagitis, biopsies, diagnosis of Barrett's esophagus, evaluate for stricture and to rule out malignancy
- A 24-hour pH monitoring of the distal esophagus to demonstrate the acid reflux

TREATMENT

Initial treatment is by medical measures.
- *Antacids:* Maalox®, Mylanta®, Pepto Bismol®
- H_2 *blockers:* Cimetidine, Zantac®
- *Proton-pump inhibitors:* Prilosec®, Nexium®, Pepcid®, Protonix®
- *Diet:* Bland diet, nonspicy food, less alcohol
- *Posture:* Semierect posture, especially after meals, is helpful
- *Lifestyle changes:* Weight reduction, small meals, walking after meals, smoking cessation, avoiding constipation or straining
- *Things to avoid:* Aspirin, nonsteroidal anti-inflammatory pain medications, big meals.

Surgery is considered when there is failure of medical treatment, if there is suspicion of malignancy, if there is evidence of Barrett's esophagus, or if there are complications such as stricture or severe esophagitis. This can be an elective procedure in the form of laparoscopic Nissen fundoplication. Various modifications of antireflux procedures are described. They strive to bring down the distal esophagus to intra-abdominal position and create a partial or complete wrap around the distal esophagus to reduce the reflux. Distal esophagectomy is considered for malignancy and Barrett's esophagus. Several antireflux procedures are being done using laparoscope, robotics, and through gastroscope. Endoscopic approaches without an incision carry some promise for the future.

KEY POINTS

Heartburn is never an emergency for surgery. Conservative therapy with medications and diet control are tried first. Failure of medical treatment, onset of complications, or suspicion of malignancy is an indication for surgical intervention.

CHAPTER 30

Obesity

INTRODUCTION

Obesity reduces life expectancy and increases morbidity. It poses special problems for the surgeon metabolically, technically, and care-wise. Obese patients are more prone to developing diabetes mellitus, respiratory complications, embolic events, cardiac complications, and wound complications. Gallstones, osteoarthritis, decubitus ulcers, thrombophlebitis, venous stasis ulcers, and hypertension are more common. Physical examination for peritoneal signs and ambulation is more difficult. Some of the investigations such as a computed tomography (CT) scan or magnetic resonance imaging (MRI) may not be possible, thus leading to a delay in diagnosis. Surgery and anesthesia pose challenges. Laparoscopic instruments and operating tables are specially ordered for them.

EVALUATION AND MANAGEMENT

Obesity is more of a problem in Western countries, whereas malnutrition is common in the developing world. Obesity reduces life expectancy by 20 years on an average, resulting from a variety of metabolic and socioeconomic problems. It comes from the habit of overeating for a long period of time and it is not easy to solve.

The physician is expected to give advice against being overweight from childhood onward. Body mass index (BMI) is calculated from height and weight, age adjusted. BMI = weight in kg/height in meter square. A BMI of over 30 kg/m^2 is a medically hazardous situation and must be treated. Calculation of BMI has been simplified with the advent of mobile phone technology, which automatically calculates the BMI once height and weight are entered.

Obese patients are at a higher risk for many medical problems such as diabetes mellitus, respiratory insufficiency, cardiac insufficiency, arthritis and joint problems, leg ulcers, hygienic issues, mental depression, decubitus ulcers, thrombophlebitis, sleep disorders, and embolic disorders. Sleep apnea syndrome and obesity hypoventilation syndrome lead to snoring, nocturnal awakening, and daytime somnolence. These items need to be addressed at all times, especially during any contemplated surgical interventions. Prophylactic measures against thromboembolic episodes with mini-dose heparin or Fragmin® are recommended. Continuous positive airway pressure (CPAP) is used for respiratory support.

Medical management is initially tried which includes advice on diet, exercises, medications, and psychosocial support. It works in motivated individuals with early onset obesity. Many different dietary regimens are available in the market with varying success. However, surgical procedures are the best options of treatment for the rest. Medications for obesity management are slowly gaining acceptance. Newer drugs such as Ozempic, Mounjaro, and Wegovy are useful for weight reduction in patients with type 2 diabetes.

Obesity management, including surgery, has proven benefits with reduction in diabetes, osteoporosis, cardiac diseases, and improvement of life expectancy. Different types of surgical procedures have been tried over a period of time. Gastric bypass with Roux-en-Y procedure, gastric banding, and intragastric balloon placement have enjoyed popularity in the last several years. However, the most recent procedure of choice appears to be the vertical sleeve gastrectomy done by the laparoscopic method or using robotic assistance. This procedure seems to have a lower complication rate and lower metabolic problems. Endoscopic methods without incisions on the skin are also gaining attention. They include intragastric balloon placement and endoscopic sleeve isolation.

Surgery needs a special table, anesthetic precautions, and special instruments. Postsurgical care needs extra attention. Wound complications are difficult to detect early and result in incisional hernia and wound dehiscence. Internal hernia, gangrene of bowel, and leak from anastomosis or gastric dilatation can occur following gastric bypass procedures.

Obesity poses challenges for the surgeon, and bariatric surgery has evolved as a subspecialty. Surgery for obesity as well as incidental surgical procedures in obese patients are challenges. Childhood and teenage obesity are becoming increasingly common. Obese patients are at a higher risk for cardiorespiratory problems, venous thrombosis, skin ulcerations, and metabolic syndromes including diabetes mellitus and create delay in clinical diagnosis and logistic problems with diagnostic tests such as MRI.

KEY POINTS

Obesity is a medical problem and must be treated. Medical treatment with diet and exercise is tried initially. Surgery is the final choice. Laparoscopic sleeve gastrectomy appears to be the procedure of choice at this time.

CHAPTER 31

Hematemesis

INTRODUCTION

Upper gastrointestinal (GI) bleeding or vomiting of blood is a scary situation. It is a horrible scene to witness someone vomiting blood, even in a small quantity. There is more panic here compared to a massive internal hemorrhage because no one sees it. It is important to differentiate true hematemesis from epistaxis and hemoptysis. Hematemesis is blood coming from the stomach or esophagus, epistaxis is blood coming from the nose or pharynx, and hemoptysis is blood coming from the trachea, bronchus, or lungs. Systemic support and investigation to find the source are done simultaneously. Once the source of bleeding is identified, efforts are taken to stop it.

FIRST STEP OF MANAGEMENT

Vomiting blood is a panic situation for the patient and family. Nursing staff and even physicians get anxious when one sees blood coming out as opposed to internal hemorrhage. Fortunately, there is always some time to think things through. First, wipe out the blood in the mouth and face and find out if it is coming from the stomach or nose. Insert a nasogastric (NG) tube and inspect the returns for blood. Inspect if it is fresh red blood or dark clotted blood. Irrigate it with cold saline to see if it is continuing or clotted already. Call for immediate consultation from the gastroenterologist and surgeon and inform the invasive radiologist to be on alert.

Initial support measures are started while efforts to diagnose and treat the problem are undertaken simultaneously. An intravenous (IV) is started and a central line inserted for reliable IV access and infusions. Blood is sent for type and crossmatch as well as for complete blood count (CBC), coagulation profile, and complete chemistry including liver chemistry. Admit the patient to the intensive care unit (ICU) or monitored bed. Examination and history may give an idea as to the etiology.

ETIOLOGY AND MANAGEMENT

- Esophageal varices
- Peptic ulcer disease
- Mallory-Weiss tear
- Acute gastritis
- Leiomyoma, carcinoma, lymphoma, polyps
- Retrograde jejunogastric intussusception.

A common problem is esophageal varices secondary to portal hypertension and cirrhosis of the liver. Usually, there is a history of alcoholism, jaundice, liver disease, prior admissions, and often ascites. These patients have end-stage liver disease. The Sengstaken-Blakemore tube had been used to provide balloon compression of the bleeding area while waiting for more definitive measures.

Esophagogastroduodenostomy (EGD) is diagnostic and therapeutic. The bleeding varices can be ligated with rubber bands or injected with sclerotherapy agents for local control. Blood transfusion and correction of coagulation abnormalities are undertaken. It is necessary to reduce portal hypertension. This is most often done by a transjugular intrahepatic portosystemic shunt (TIPS) procedure, which is done by the interventional radiologist. Various types of portosystemic shunts were done in the past, most of which have been abandoned with the advent of the noninvasive procedure of TIPS. In the TIPS procedure, a stent is placed over a guidewire, via the internal jugular vein, threading it through the vena cava, through the hepatic vein, through the parenchyma of the liver, and into a large branch of the portal vein.

A second common etiology is peptic ulcer disorders. The incidence has come down with the use of H_2 blockers and proton pump inhibitors. Another reason could be acute gastritis, Mallory-Weiss tear of distal esophageal mucosa, or distal esophagitis. Again, a history of the intake of nonsteroidal pain medications, history of peptic ulcer disease, and hiatal hernia may give clues. An urgent EGD can be both diagnostic and therapeutic. The site of bleeding and cause of bleeding can be identified, and endoscopic treatments are undertaken at the same time. This could be by injection of epinephrine, cauterization of the bleeding area, or application of clips. Persistent bleeding can be further studied and treated by selective angiogram and embolization.

The last resort is to do open surgery, to suture ligate the bleeding area, and to do acid-reducing procedures if necessary. At surgery after laparotomy, the stomach is opened toward the area where the bleeding was emanating, based on endoscopy. Clots are quickly evacuated and the stomach is packed to expose the bleeding site. Once the actual bleeding spot or spurting vessel is identified, the area is securely suture ligated with silk sutures in a figure-of-eight fashion. The first priority is to stop the bleeding. After this has been accomplished, additional steps can be considered to reduce future bleeding. For example, this may involve doing a pyloroplasty and vagotomy in the case of a large penetrating posterior duodenal ulcer or doing a partial gastrectomy for an ulcerated leiomyoma. Gastric ulcers are likely to be malignant; therefore, a gastrectomy is preferable in treating gastric ulcers. A biopsy of the edges of the ulcer is done along with suture ligation of the bleeding area. Bleeding from the Mallory–Weiss tear from the distal esophagus is sutured under vision. This tear involves the mucosa of the distal esophagus as a result of excessive vomiting or trauma from an NG tube.

Medical management of the underlying disease is equally important with the use of antacids, H_2 blockers, proton-pump inhibitors, thiamin, vitamin K, tranexamic acid, and nutritional support.

Less common causes of hematemesis are cancers, polyps, leiomyoma, lymphoma, and retrograde jejunogastric intussusception **(Box 31.1)**. An endoscopy is a good diagnostic starting point, with treatment directed according to the specific situation. Vascular malformation of the stomach is known as Dieulafoy lesion and can often be treated with endoscopic sclerotherapy.

An interventional radiologist can be of great assistance in diagnosing the source of bleeding and treating it. They can do a selective angiogram to find the source of bleeding and inject coils or gel foam to embolize the specific artery. Hemobilia is a condition where blood seeps into the common bile duct (CBD) from the liver following trauma to the liver, where the interventional radiologist is especially helpful to selectively occlude the branch of hepatic artery.

An aortoduodenal fistula is a rare postaortic surgery complication where the aortic graft erodes into the duodenum resulting in massive upper GI hemorrhage. A vascular surgeon is consulted for emergency surgery. Ideally, the aorta is crossclamped at the hiatus, the area of adhesion between the duodenum and aortic graft is separated, and the holes in the graft and duodenum are repaired securely. The area is profusely irrigated, closed with a patch of omentum in between the organs, and given IV antibiotics.

Subsequently, the decision is made to take down this aortic graft and do extra-anatomic bypass to avoid bacteremia, mycotic aneurysm formation, and recurrent massive bleeding or sepsis.

> **BOX 31.1:** Hematemesis.
>
> - *First steps:* Start good IV, consider central line placement, NG tube placement, blood work to include complete blood count, type and crossmatch, coagulation profile, and liver chemistry
> - *Identify source and cause of bleeding:* Esophageal varices, peptic ulcer, Mallory–Weiss tear, cancers, leiomyoma
> - *Tests:* Upper GI endoscopy is diagnostic and therapeutic—can clip, inject, coagulate, ligate
> - Interventional radiologist can identify and embolize bleeding spot
> - TIPS procedure for portal hypertension
> - *Surgery:* Final definitive step to stop the bleeding by suturing or resecting the bleeding area, or open portosystemic bypass procedures for portal hypertension
> - *Medical:* H_2 blockers, proton pump inhibitors, antacids, and somatostatin
>
> (GI: gastrointestinal; IV: intravenous; NG: nasogastric; TIPS: transjugular intrahepatic portosystemic shunt)

KEY POINTS

Do not panic. Send blood for type and crossmatch; do CBC, liver chemistry, and prothrombin time (PT) and partial thromboplastin time (PTT). Call your gastroenterologist for EGD. Alert your surgeon. Transfer to ICU and monitor. Specific treatments will follow according to GI recommendations. Surgery will be needed if endoscopic measures fail to achieve control of bleeding. The exact nature of surgery will depend upon the etiology and source of bleeding. An interventional radiologist can be of assistance in identifying the source of bleeding and at times in controlling the bleeding by selective embolization of the bleeding artery.

# SECTION 4

Anorectal Conditions

32. Bleeding Per Rectum
33. Pain in the Anal Region
34. Hemorrhoids
35. Prolapse of the Rectum
36. Pruritus Ani
37. Pilonidal Cyst
38. Carcinoma of Colon and Rectum

CHAPTER 32

Bleeding Per Rectum

INTRODUCTION

Lower gastrointestinal (GI) bleeding can be sudden and massive or slow and chronic, to the extent that the patient presents with anemia. It can be fresh red blood coming from the anal margin, such as hemorrhoidal bleed, or burgundy color coming from the upper rectum or sigmoid colon, such as diverticular disease. Occasionally, it can be coming from the postpyloric area with a rapid transit through the bowels. The critical step is to find the source of bleeding. Sometimes, this is easy and at other times it can be very challenging. Rectal cancer and colon cancer must be ruled out in all cases of rectal bleeding.

FIRST STEP OF MANAGEMENT

Assess the severity of bleeding and vital signs. If it is massive or recurrent, admit the patient, start intravenous (IV), send blood for type and match, and do routine blood tests including complete blood count (CBC), coagulation profile, and liver chemistry. Examine the patient, do a rectal examination, and look at the type of stool or blood on the examining finger.

ETIOLOGY AND MANAGEMENT

If it is painful, it can be anal in origin. Painless bleeding arises from above the dentate line. If it is massive, it could be coming from the rectum or higher up. Slow bleeding is from the lower anus.

Fresh red blood unmixed with stool is from the anal margin. When it is mixed with stool or is burgundy in color, it means that it is coming from the rectum or higher up in the colon.

A simple bedside proctoscopic examination will show anal hemorrhoids and fissure. Stool in the rectum can be inspected to see if it is clear brown or mixed with blood. On rare occasions, massive upper GI bleeding from the area distal to the pylorus can present as rectal bleeding. Insert a nasogastric (NG) tube to see if there is any blood in the stomach.

The most common cause of bleeding from the anal margin is hemorrhoids. This can be seen and diagnosed with proctoscopy. The best treatment is to do a hemorrhoidectomy with suture ligation of the bleeding areas.

The most common cause of colonic bleeding is diverticular disease. Most of them are in the sigmoid colon, but they can be spread throughout the colon. Bleeding from the right colon or cecum can fill the entire colon, whereas bleeding from the sigmoid colon usually leaves the right colon free of blood, with blood only in the left colon.

Angiodysplasia usually involves the cecum and the blood can fill the entire colon. Rarely, the small bowel can be the source of bleeding, such as Meckel's diverticulum, diverticula, cancers, and polyps. Colitis of different types such as ulcerative colitis, Crohn's colitis, infectious colitis, and ischemic colitis can also cause bleeding. They can be a challenge to diagnose accurately.

TESTS AND CONSULTATIONS

Consult a gastroenterologist for colonoscopic evaluation. Even in situations of active bleeding, the examination is helpful to know if the bleeding is from the left colon, right colon, or higher up. Usually, they do an upper and lower endoscopy for completion sake.

A bleeding nuclear scan can show the severity of bleeding and the general location of the bleeding area. A selective angiogram is both diagnostic and therapeutic in situations of massive bleeding.

TREATMENT

Massive painless bleeding per rectum is usually due to diverticulitis. The blood is often initially mixed with stool and is somewhat burgundy in color. There can be multiple profuse bleeding episodes enough to warrant admission and blood transfusion. A rectal examination will show that the stool is mixed with blood, indicating that the bleeding is coming from higher up than the anal margin, probably from the sigmoid colon. A colonoscopy may not reveal the actual site of bleeding but will give an idea as to which side of the colon is bleeding and the etiology, such as diverticular disease or cancer.

Fortunately, most lower GI bleeding stops spontaneously. If the bleeding remains persistent, or if the patient requires more than six units of blood transfusion, surgery is done. This will most commonly involve resection of the segment of colon that is the culprit and anastomosis at the same sitting. At times, there are diverticula all over the colon and it is difficult to know the actual site or side of bleeding. In these instances, it is better to do a subtotal colectomy with ileorectal anastomosis.

Angiodysplasia is often from the cecal region. A bleeding scan while the patient is actively bleeding can also help to know the general location of bleeding. A selective angiogram can also be helpful. If the bleeding spots can be effectively coagulated at colonoscopy, then the patient can be observed. If it is unsuccessful, then a right hemicolectomy is done.

Fresh bright red blood per rectum, unmixed with stool, at the time of defecation is often hemorrhoids. The bleeding is also painless and splatters the toilet basin. A rectal examination will show brown stool in the rectal ampulla and an anal examination will show the hemorrhoids. They may require surgery or rubber band ligation.

Carcinoma of rectum must be ruled out in all cases of rectal bleeding **(Box 32.1)**. Usually, the bleeding is intermittent and in small amounts. Rectal examination, proctoscopy, and sigmoidoscopy are done to make sure that there is no malignancy in the rectum or lower sigmoid colon. If carcinoma of colon or rectum is diagnosed, the first choice is to do multidisciplinary oncological evaluation. Staging of the cancer, evaluation of metastasis, and risk factors are done. Minimally invasive procedures are considered first. Radical surgery may be needed as the best chance for cure. This may involve abdominoperineal resection (APR), total mesorectal excision (TME), or colectomy. Patients are appropriately staged with workup. They may need adjuvant radiation or chemotherapy per protocols.

A small amount of bleeding associated with pain on defecation is usually seen in fissure-in-ano or fistulae.

There are instances where the patient bleeds intermittently, but most tests come back as negative. This can be frustrating and challenging, requiring multiple admissions and transfusions. Small bowel evaluation with capsule endoscopy, selective angiogram with venous phase study of superior and inferior mesenteric arteries, red cell tagged scans, and technetium scan are options. Ultimately, open laparotomy has been done to thoroughly explore the small bowel and the rest of the GI tract.

KEY POINTS

Do not ignore rectal bleeding. Make sure that there is no rectal cancer. Lower GI bleeding can be initially treated by supportive measures since it stops spontaneously.

BOX 32.1: Causes and treatment of lower gastrointestinal bleeding.

- Fresh red blood unmixed with stool is probably hemorrhoidal or anal margin pathology
- Maroon color blood mixed with stool is probably diverticular or sigmoid colon pathology
- *Tests:* Proctosigmoidoscopy, colonoscopy, gastrografin enema, computed tomography (CT) scan, nuclear bleeding scan, selective angiogram
- *Treatment:* Most bleedings stop spontaneously. When the bleeding continues, surgical intervention is needed. Sigmoid colectomy, extended left colectomy, subtotal colectomy, right colectomy, and hemorrhoidectomy are options depending on the exact situation

CHAPTER 33: Pain in the Anal Region

INTRODUCTION

Extreme pain in the perianal region is an emergency and is usually sudden in onset. Careful examination of the anal and perianal region will reveal etiology such as fissure-in-ano, thrombosed external hemorrhoid, or perianal abscess. Sometimes, this could be due to trauma or skin infections. The patient may have other chronic conditions such as condyloma or carcinoma and may seek evaluation as a painful condition.

EVALUATION AND MANAGEMENT

Severe pain in the perianal region of short duration is usually due to one of the following three conditions: (1) Acute fissure-in-ano; (2) Thrombosed external hemorrhoids; or (3) Perianal abscess.

Fissure-in-ano is basically a tear of the anal mucosa. Since this part of the anal canal is ectodermal in origin, it has somatic sensory nervous supply **(Box 33.1)**. Constipation, straining, or a hard stool could cause it. Acute fissures may be associated with a small amount of rectal bleeding, blood being seen as a line along one side of the stool. Inspection of the anal mucosa by retraction of the area will reveal the tear. The patient will refuse a rectal examination because of the pain **(Fig. 33.1)**.

Treatments involve sitz baths, stool softeners, and topical application of Xylocaine® jelly mixed with a small amount of nitroglycerine to relax the anal sphincter. Botox injections help to relieve anal spasm.

Chronic fissures of long-standing nature have a scar tissue at the base of the fissure. These patients may require fissurectomy and sphincterotomy either through the base of the fissure or by lateral sphincterotomy.

In certain chronic fissures, especially occurring in lateral positions, one should be aware of etiological factors such as human immunodeficiency virus (HIV)/acquired immunodeficiency syndrome (AIDS), syphilis, tuberculosis, and Crohn's disease.

Thrombosed external hemorrhoid is a sudden bleeding into an external hemorrhoid skin tag. It is usually a venous bleeding and presents as painful swelling at the anal margin, often with a bluish-red appearance. It is painful because it involves a sudden stretching of the skin and ectodermal tissue. In the early phase, it can be treated by an incision and evacuation of the hematoma, also known as enucleation of the external thrombotic hemorrhoid. Once it is organized and edematous, it will need to be excised.

Perianal abscess is an infectious process. It often starts as a cryptoglandular infection in the anal area. It can occur at the anal margin, intersphincteric, or ischiorectal region **(Box 33.2)**. Severe pain associated with fever and leukocytosis, often with a swelling or boggy appearance, is noted.

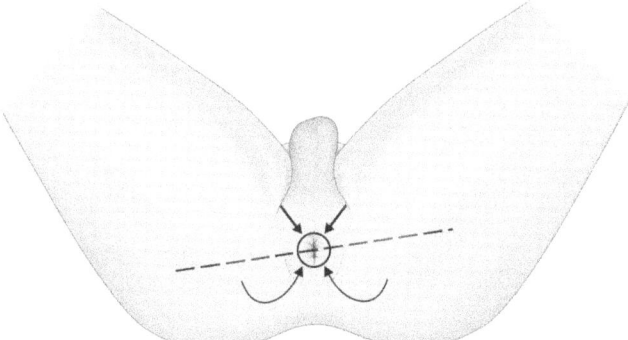

- Anterior fistula is short and straight
- Posterior fistula takes a curve path to open in midline posteriorly

Fig. 33.1: Fistula-in-ano—Goodsall's rule.

BOX 33.1: Causes and treatment of *fissure-in-ano*.

Causes:
- It is a tear of the anal mucosa, which causes pain
- Patient refuses rectal examination due to pain

Treatment: Acute phase—dietary advice, sitz baths, avoiding constipation, stool softeners, Xylocaine® jelly with nitroglycerine, botox injection. Chronic phase—fissurectomy, sphincterotomy

> **BOX 33.2:** Symptoms, tests, and treatment of perianal abscess.
>
> - *Symptoms:* Pain, swelling, and discomfort in the perianal region with fever, leukocytosis of short duration, progressively worsening
> - *Tests:* Sonogram, pelvic computed tomography (CT) scan, bedside needle aspiration. Physical examination is enough most of the time
> - *Treatment:*
>   – Incision and drainage in the operating room, adequate size incision, wound left open with packing
>   – Intravenous (IV) antibiotics, wound cultures
>   – At surgery, make sure that there is no fistula-in-ano
>   – At surgery, make sure that there is no extension to the opposite side or to the ischiorectal area

One may not elicit a fluctuation in these cases. A perianal ultrasound or a computed tomography (CT) scan could help. A needle aspiration at the bedside is also an option.

These patients need wide incision, drainage, and debridement in the operating room under anesthesia. At surgery, it is important to make sure that the abscess cavity is completely opened up and explored and to make sure that there is no fistula-in-ano as a causative factor. The wound is packed and left open for proper drainage and intravenous (IV) antibiotics are given.

Other causes of pain in the anal region are fistula-in-ano, proctalgia fugax, proctitis induced by inflammatory bowel diseases, infections, radiation therapy, and acute trauma.

In fistula-in-ano, there is an abnormal communication between the anal canal and the exterior skin, which can open and close periodically, can be a source of pain or recurrent infection, and can lead to drainage of feculent material through the sinus tract. Usually, it is resultant of a crypt abscess that ruptures to the exterior. Rare causes can be lymphogranuloma venerium. The fistula is explored and probed in the operating room, and it is laid open completely, and the wound is allowed to heal by secondary intention. If the fistula is a high fistula with the internal opening above the anal sphincter, care is taken to avoid dividing through the sphincter in one stage for fear of causing incontinence of stool. In such situations, a seton is used to divide the sphincter in stages.

Proctalgia fugax is a poorly understood condition, where transient fleeting sharp pain is felt in the anal region. This is related to pelvic pathologies, prostatitis, urinary bladder, or vaginal infections.

Proctitis is inflammation of the rectum. This is related to inflammatory bowel disorders, bacterial infections, or radiation therapy to pelvic areas. Application of Vaseline or steroid creams may be of help, along with sitz bath.

Acute trauma to the anal region can happen following instrumentation, severe constipation, or anal sex activities.

KEY POINTS

Severe pain in the anal region is usually due to:
- Acute fissure-in-ano
- Thrombosed external hemorrhoid
- Perianal abscess

CHAPTER 34

Hemorrhoids

INTRODUCTION

Hemorrhoids are a commonly used terminology to describe protrusions at the anal canal. While the external hemorrhoids are loose skin tags, the internal hemorrhoids are engorged vascular columns under the anal mucosa. Bleeding is a common symptom. However, they can be prolapsing, thrombosed, and inflamed masses creating a painful and difficult situation that can be corrected only by surgery. They can become more prominent due to portal hypertension, cirrhosis of the liver, pelvic tumors, pregnancy, or vena cava obstruction.

Patients often refer to any anal or perianal problems as "I have hemorrhoids." The physician has to make the diagnosis of hemorrhoids by inspection, palpation, a rectal examination, and proctoscopic examination along with the history given by the patient. There are no tests needed here. Always make sure that a rectal cancer is not missed, since patients can refer to all rectal problems as hemorrhoids.

EXTERNAL HEMORRHOIDS

External hemorrhoids are just skin tags outside the dentate line, covered by ectodermal tissue. The patient notices protruding tissue that is made of skin and subcutaneous tissue, with occasional itching or discomfort and hygienic issues. Suddenly, they can develop a blood clot inside from a ruptured vein. Then it becomes very painful, presenting as a small cherry at the anal margin. The best treatment at this early phase is to inject local anesthetic, incise over it, and evacuate the blood clot. It is also called "enucleation of external thrombotic hemorrhoids." Sometimes, these get completely thrombosed, presenting as large, painful, nonreducible masses. In these situations, they have to be excised completely.

INTERNAL HEMORRHOIDS

Internal hemorrhoids are engorged veins in the submucosa, above the dentate line. Initially, they are asymptomatic. Painless, fresh red blood unmixed with stool is the telltale symptom when the veins rupture and bleed. Straining and constipation aggravate this. Subsequently, they can get larger and start prolapsing. They are graded depending upon the extent of prolapse: Grade 1—with no prolapse, grade 2—small prolapse with spontaneous reduction, grade 3—prolapse that needs manual reduction, and grade 4—nonreducible prolapse.

Hemorrhoids can become more prominent and prolapsing when there is increased venous pressure in the pelvic veins and in situations such as portal hypertension, cirrhosis of the liver, pelvic tumors, pregnancy, and vena cava obstruction.

Medical treatment is recommended for first- and second-degree hemorrhoids. A diet that reduces constipation and increases bulk soft stool is recommended. This includes vegetables, fruits, fluids, fiber, and avoidance of red meat. No strains for bowel movements with regular bowel habits are aimed for. Stool softener medications, such as Surfak® and Colace®, or stool bulk-forming medications, such as Metamucil, are useful.

Office procedures without surgery can be considered for first- and second-degree hemorrhoids. These include injection of sclerosing agents to the base of the hemorrhoid, rubber band ligation of the hemorrhoids, or infrared coagulation of the hemorrhoidal base.

Surgical treatment is the ultimate choice for third- and fourth-degree hemorrhoids and for complicated hemorrhoids, such as prolapsed and thrombosed ones. The hemorrhoidal pedicle is isolated and securely ligated after dissecting out the hemorrhoidal mass. The mucocutaneous junction is approximated to reduce pain, reduce anal stricture, and promote faster healing. External hemorrhoidal tissues can be incorporated in the excision. Care is taken to retain adequate anoderm between hemorrhoidal excisions to minimize the chance of anal stenosis. Use of staples to do a stapled hemorrhoidectomy has gained attention. It is also known as procedure for prolapsed hemorrhoid (PPH). A circular stapling device is used to remove a ring of tissue from the prolapsed hemorrhoid. This reduces the blood supply to the hemorrhoid and lifts it back. The procedure is not suitable for all and can have its own technical complications.

KEY POINTS

External hemorrhoids are just skin tags with loose skin. Internal hemorrhoids are engorged veins in the anal submucosa that can bleed. Patients refer to all anorectal problems as hemorrhoids. It is up to the physician to make the correct diagnosis by doing a proper examination.

CHAPTER 35

Prolapse of the Rectum

INTRODUCTION

Prolapse of the rectum is a protrusion of tissue outside the anal margin. True prolapse of the rectum, also known as procidentia, is a full thick eversion of the rectal wall with circumferential mucosa exposed outside. This has to be differentiated from prolapse of hemorrhoids or polyps. Three factors contribute for the procidentia to happen: (1) Weak pelvic floor as seen in elderly or neurologically deficient patients; (2) Very redundant sigmoid colon mesentery; and (3) Very weak and patulous anal sphincter with low strength of the sphincter muscle.

PROLAPSE

Every so often a patient states that there is a protrusion from the anal margin. At times, it is the caregiver of an elderly patient or the mother of a child who makes the observation.

Prolapse can involve anal mucosa only, which retracts spontaneously after a bowel movement, or it can be a full-thickness protrusion of the whole wall reversing inside out. This full-thickness prolapse is actually an intussusception at the anal margin.

Large prolapsed thrombosed hemorrhoids remaining nonreducible are at times mistaken for prolapse of the rectum. Such fourth-degree hemorrhoids require excision and hemorrhoidectomy.

Large full-thickness true prolapse of the rectum is due to three basic pathophysiology issues: (1) Very weak pelvic floor; (2) Patulous and weak anal sphincter; and (3) Redundant sigmoid mesentery. Hence, these three aspects should be addressed during the surgical repair.

Conditions that predispose prolapse of rectum include senility, dementia, pregnancy, childhood, neurological disorders, multiparity, multiple vaginal deliveries, female sex, chronic straining, and pelvic floor defects.

Medical management includes advice to avoid constipation, avoid straining, pelvic floor exercises to strengthen the anal sphincter and pelvic muscles, and to keep the prolapse tissue reduced manually to avoid bleeding and excoriation.

Surgery is the definitive treatment. Old techniques such as Thiersch wire or nylon suturing around the anus have been abandoned. The current surgery procedure recommends an abdominal approach or a perineal approach. The Altemeier technique involving perineal proctosigmoidectomy from the anal margin is a very effective procedure that can be done under spinal anesthesia and is well tolerated by elderly patients. There is no abdominal incision and the anastomosis is at the anal margin after perineal pull-through. An alternative procedure is an abdominal proctosigmoidectomy with the placement of a Marlex® mesh to perform proctopexy as done in the Ripstein procedure. In both cases, efforts must be made to suture the weakened levator muscles.

Newer techniques are: (1) Transanal total mesorectal excision (TaTME), where laparoscopic and special instruments are used for resection of the prolapsed segment transanal; (2) Improved robotic techniques, which are used for proctopexy through minimally invasive procedures; and (3) Injection of bulking agents to tissues around the rectum to provide support.

KEY POINTS

Prolapsed thrombosed inflamed hemorrhoids need to be differentiated from true prolapse of rectum, which is in effect an anal intussusception.

CHAPTER 36

Pruritus Ani

INTRODUCTION

Many patients with anorectal disorders present with symptoms of anal and perianal itching. The underlying cause could be benign conditions such as pinworm infestation and condyloma or could be a malignant condition such as squamous cell carcinoma. A careful physical examination, rectal examination, and proctoscopic examination can reveal the exact problem. Biopsies may be necessary at times. Treatment is directed to the underlying etiology.

ETIOLOGY

An itching and scratching sensation in the anal and perianal region can be an annoying symptom.

Common causes are pinworm or other helminthic infestations, condyloma acuminata, sphincteric incontinence, and anal hygiene.

PINWORM

Pinworm infestation is common in tropical countries. It is from contaminated food intake. As the patient scratches the anal region, the eggs of the worm are transmitted to the person's mouth from the fingernails, creating a new cycle of infestation. Stool examination may show the worm itself or the eggs. Albendazole or mebendazole is good for all parasitic infestations.

CONDYLOMA

Examination of the anal area will reveal anal warts, which are usually due to condyloma. Patients will often confirm having homosexual contacts and may have associated human immunodeficiency virus (HIV) infections. The warts themselves are caused by human papillomavirus (HPV) and have no curative treatment. They can be very small and isolated or large and confluent.

Condylomas are best treated with complete excision and fulguration in the operating room. They will require repeat sittings of similar fulgurations because of a high chance of recurrences. The mode of excision can be by electrocautery, by cryotherapy, or by using lasers. Smoke evacuation is mandatory in these cases while doing the procedure.

Topical application of medications is also described. These include podophyllin, trichloroacetic acid, 5-fluorouracil, and imiquimod 5% cream. There is a 30–40% chance of recurrence irrespective of the type of treatment. Hence, close monitoring and repeat treatment sessions are needed.

INCONTINENCE AND ANAL HYGIENE

Incomplete cleansing of the anal area after bowel movements or anal incontinence leaves moisture and particles, which can lead to an itching sensation. Hygienic precautions and sphincteric exercises are recommended. Medications to reduce transit time, antidiarrheals, and anticholinergics have been tried. Surgical repairs with sphincter reconstruction and sphincteroplasty are done for intractable cases.

Other causes of perianal itching can be due to prolapse of anal mucosa, fistula-in-ano, hidradenitis suppurativa, and sexually transmitted disorders. Malignant disorders of anorectum such as squamous cell carcinoma, Paget's disease, and basal cell carcinoma can also cause an itching sensation. Biopsy of the lesion is required for a definitive diagnosis. They can spread to inguinal lymph nodes or deep iliac lymph nodes.

KEY POINTS

Perianal itching can be due to condyloma acuminata, pinworm infestation, or soiling of the anal area due to poor hygiene or anal incontinence. However, any other anorectal problems including cancers can have an itching sensation as the first presenting symptom. Hence, careful examination is needed in all cases.

CHAPTER 37

Pilonidal Cyst

INTRODUCTION

Pilonidal cyst is a condition that results in infection in the presacral coccygeal area of young individuals with hair in the area. They present with recurrent draining sinuses and abscesses or painful spots in this region. Close examination will show one to three small pinhole openings in the skin at the midline coccygeal area. If they are probed under anesthesia, a tunnel for varying distances under the skin can be detected. These tunnels have hair and lint sucked into them.

DIAGNOSIS AND TREATMENT

Patients are usually young adults who present with inflammation or draining focus in the presacral region. The word "pilus" means hair and "nidus" means nest, meaning a nest for hairballs. It reveals the causative factor in the pathophysiology of the condition. Risk factors for the condition include the presence of excessive hair in the posterior presacral area, obesity, a sedentary lifestyle, deep natal cleft, and family history.

One or more small punctums or holes occur in the midline of presacral/coccygeal skin. It is thought to be a congenital defect from the fusion of two sides of the body. Once this hole is formed, hair, lint, and dirt get pulled into it due to the bellow-like suction effect from the two buttocks. A tunnel is formed under the skin for varying lengths. The mouth of the tract gets plugged with the materials such as hair or lint, which leads to infection and abscess formation.

Physical examination shows these holes in the midline, over the tailbone. They are not located in the perirectal area, but well above it over the coccygeal area. One to three midline tiny holes can be seen on the skin. An abscess is noted above or to one side of these holes. They may give a history of prior abscess that has been drained. Sometimes, these abscesses burst spontaneously leaving sinus tracts with external openings connecting to the midline holes.

If there is an acute abscess, it has to be drained for immediate relief. Making a direct incision over the most prominent part of the abscess is appropriate. In addition to pus, one may see hair follicles and dirt material in the abscess. Antibiotics are given to counteract the infection. After the infection has subsided, a more definitive surgery is done to prevent recurrence.

Uninfected pilonidal cysts need elective surgery to excise the pilonidal cyst. An elliptical incision is made vertically to remove the skin holes and the subcutaneous tissue down to the presacral fascia. Good hemostasis is obtained. The wound can be packed lightly and the skin closed to avoid leaving a large open wound. Otherwise, it can be left open for secondary closure. Another option is called marsupialization, where the tract is simply laid open and the epithelialized tracts freshened. Recurrence is a possibility. Complex pilonidal cysts with recurrent large tracts need wider excisions, followed by flap closures.

KEY POINTS

Diagnosis is to be made from other skin infections and perianal abscesses by the specific location and skin holes in the midline coccygeal area.

CHAPTER 38

Carcinoma of Colon and Rectum

INTRODUCTION

Colorectal cancers are common and require special awareness and recognition in the daily activities of the general surgeon. If diagnosed and treated early, there is hope for a better outcome. There has been much progress in this field during the past few years.

DIAGNOSIS

A good number of cases are now detected on routine screening colonoscopy before they become symptomatic. The current recommendation is to do routine annual screening colonoscopy from the age of 40 till the age of 75 years. This is because of the finding of increasing colon cancers in the adult population. Moreover, many polyps are discovered incidentally, excised, and biopsied. A routine rectal examination during every physical examination and hemoccult testing of the stool also leads to further investigation and diagnosis.

Stool examinations for occult blood and cancer cells are available tools for early detection. Cologuard test for deoxyribonucleic acid (DNA) analysis of the stool for cancer cells and fecal immunoassay test (FIT) are such tests.

Symptoms noted by the patient may include alteration of bowel habits, change in caliber of the stool, blood in the stool, burgundy and dark-colored stool, abdominal pain, cramps, unexplained weight loss, and symptoms of indigestion. Physical examination may show a palpable mass in the abdomen or enlarged liver.

ETIOLOGY AND PREVENTION

A diet high in hydrocarbons, red meat, processed food, and low residue diet are considered as contributing factors for colorectal cancers. Polyps of all varieties are predisposing conditions, more so with villous adenomas. Genetic predisposition is a proven risk factor.

Routine screening colonoscopy has a preventive role, by removing small polyps, which can turn malignant. Routine stool tests as described above can lead to colonoscopy.

INVESTIGATIONS

Biopsy proof of malignancy is recommended in all cases. Punch biopsy of palpable low-lying rectal cancers can be done as an office procedure. Lesions higher up will need a colonoscopic or sigmoidoscopic biopsy.

Virtual colonoscopy is an option for initial screening. It has the advantage of being noninvasive but has the disadvantage of false readings and need for follow-up regular colonoscopy if any abnormalities are identified.

Once a diagnosis of cancer is made, the next step is to stage the disease, whether it is confined to mucosa alone (Dukes A) or gone through full thickness of the wall (Dukes B), gone through the wall and to the regional lymph nodes (Dukes C), or has spread to distant organs by metastasis (Dukes D).

Endoscopic ultrasound is helpful in this process, along with computed tomography (CT) scan of the abdomen, regional focused magnetic resonance imaging (MRI) scan, and positive emission tomography (PET) scan. Multidisciplinary tumor board discussion with a review of all the tests is helpful.

TREATMENT

Surgery is still the mainstay of treatment. Adjuvant therapy includes radiation therapy and chemotherapy. Treatment can be curative or palliative. Newer protocols and modalities of treatment have shown improved results. Surgery can be done by different methods, open approach in a conventional way, in a laparoscopic or laparoscopic hand-assisted way, or in a robotic-assisted way.

For Dukes A lesion, the first line of treatment is radical surgery to remove the segment of the colon with regional lymph nodes. This may involve right hemicolectomy for lesions affecting the cecum, appendix, ascending colon, and hepatic flexure. Ileocolic and right colic arteries are ligated at the base, in order to remove the regional lymph nodes. Primary end-to-end anastomosis of the bowel ends from terminal ileum to mid-transverse colon is performed. For lesions involving splenic flexure, descending colon, and proximal sigmoid colon, a left hemicolectomy is done with ligation of the left colic artery at the base and anastomosing the transverse colon to the sigmoid colon.

For lesions involving the sigmoid colon, sigmoid resection is often adequate if the inferior mesenteric artery can be ligated at its base. End-to-end anastomosis will require complete mobilization of splenic flexure.

For cancers involving the upper rectum, surgery can be done by doing a low anterior resection. The resection will require mobilization of the rectum, and anastomosis can be done using EEA™ (end to end anastomosis) stapler device. The procedure can be done by open method, laparoscopic hand-assisted method, or robotic-assisted method. For good cancer clearance surgery, the procedure of total mesorectal excision (TME) is done, where the inferior mesenteric artery is ligated at the origin, and clearance of all perirectal fat and lymph nodes is done.

Cancers involving the lower rectum are evaluated carefully as to the staging. If they are Dukes A lesions, all efforts are now being made for endorectal resection of the cancer, using special endorectal instruments and robotics to avoid an abdominoperineal resection with permanent colostomy. Additional adjuvant chemotherapy and radiation therapy are considered before or after surgery. If they are Dukes B or C stages, preoperative adjuvant chemotherapy and radiation are given followed by radical cancer surgery that will involve abdominoperineal resection. Dukes D lesions with distant metastasis are treated with systemic chemotherapy. The most suitable palliative surgery for the primary lesion is considered.

Cancers of the anal canal below the dentate line are usually squamous cell cancers. They are treated with initial radiation therapy and chemotherapy followed by wide excision of the primary. The spread of this cancer is to inguinal or external iliac lymph nodes. They may need radical groin dissection if there is evidence of metastasis to these nodes.

If there is evidence of solitary metastasis to the liver, with no other evidence of metastasis on various investigations, then a partial liver resection is done followed by chemotherapy. If there is more than one spot of metastasis all confined to one lobe of the liver, then resection of that lobe is justified. For other metastatic spots in the liver, attempts to control the disease are done using infrared coagulation, cryotherapy or local excision or regional hepatic artery perfusion of chemotherapy agents. Aggressive treatment of colorectal malignancies is justified because of better chances of longevity.

KEY POINTS

Early diagnosis of colorectal cancers gives better chance for cure. Multidisciplinary approach gives better results. Recent trends show younger adults are also susceptible to get colon cancers.

SECTION 5

Head and Neck

39. Epistaxis
40. Mass in Front of the Neck: Thyroid
41. Thyroglossal Duct Cyst
42. Mass on Side of Neck: Lymph Nodes

CHAPTER 39

Epistaxis

INTRODUCTION

Epistaxis is bleeding from the nose. The most common cause is bleeding from anterior nares, secondary to trauma. This can be easily controlled by the application of local pressure. Bleeding from the posterior nasal area and nasopharynx can be very problematic. One will have to rule out carcinoma or bleeding diathesis. Posterior nasal packing is done combined with anterior nasal packing. Epistaxis of significant severity can be life-threatening and can be mistaken for hemoptysis.

ETIOLOGY

The most common cause of nasal bleeding is from some sort of trauma. It could be just picking the nose with sharp nail or some instruments. It could result from a fight, punch on the face, or fall, resulting in fracture of the nasal bone. Surgery involving maxillary sinus or other paranasal sinuses can result in postoperative bleeding from the nose. Insertion of stiff nasogastric tubes and nasotracheal tubes can cause trauma. Dry air weather, allergies, nasal congestion from any reason, irritation by exposure to flumes, and smokes can cause epistaxis. High blood pressure, hematological disorders such as hemophilia, Von Willebrand disease, and thrombocytopenia are to be ruled out. Medications such as anticoagulants, antiplatelet agents, and nonsteroidal anti-inflammatory agents can initiate bleeding.

DIAGNOSIS AND TREATMENT

Bleeding from the nose can be very alarming and disconcerting to the patient and family. It is commonly seen in children and is coming from the front of the nose due to trauma related to picking the nose with finger, nails, or other objects. The patient is asked to keep the head down and apply firm compression over the nose. Nasal packing of the anterior nose is done for persistent bleeding. At times, the packing may have to be left in place for 1-3 days. Use of topical hemostatic agents in the form of powder, gel, or patches enhances hemostasis with packing.

However, bleeding from the posterior nares can be more serious and related to congestion of the nasal mucosa. One must rule out malignancies, nasopharyngeal carcinoma, or angiomas. Other possibilities are bleeding disorders such as leukemia, hemophilia, hypertension, and excessive anticoagulation. Head injuries and fractures of the nasal bones related to trauma must be elicited by history. Hematological and bleeding disorders, metastatic malignancies, immunecompromised conditions, and intracranial tumors are held in differential diagnosis.

Posterior nasal packing is done to stop the posterior nasal bleeding. Sometimes, a Foley catheter is placed, and the balloon is inflated. Coagulation factors are corrected. The packing may have to be left in place for 3 days. Nasal packing with expandable sponges and inflatable balloons is a helpful measure. Use of electrocautery or lasers under anesthesia is sometimes needed. If still unsuccessful, interventional radiology may help to identify the bleeding area and do selective embolization. Ligation of external carotid artery or sphenopalatine artery can be done.

Hemoptysis and hematemesis can be mistaken for nasal bleeding and must be differentiated by proper examination. In addition to the nasal packing, care to avoid airway obstruction and aspiration pneumonia is undertaken.

Complete blood count and coagulation profiles are checked. If necessary, a computed tomography (CT) scan or magnetic resonance imaging (MRI) of the head and sinuses is obtained.

KEY POINTS

Most nasal bleeding is due to local trauma and can be controlled by local tamponade.

CHAPTER 40

Mass in Front of the Neck: Thyroid

INTRODUCTION

Enlargement of the thyroid is called a goiter. Thyroid masses make up most of the masses in the front of the neck. Occasionally, other soft-tissue masses can be present in this location. The two main issues regarding thyroid are: (1) to know if it is functioning as a hyperactive or hypoactive organ and (2) to know if the given mass is cancerous or benign. With these goals, one should do thyroid function tests and sonogram-guided fine needle aspiration (FNA) cytology in all thyroid masses. If the thyroid is hyperactive, as in Graves' disease, then antithyroid medications are given. If it is hypoactive, as in myxedema, then thyroid supplements are given. If there is any suspicion of malignancy in the FNA, it is best to plan for a total thyroidectomy. If it is a benign goiter, one may treat it with partial thyroidectomy or with thyroid suppression therapy, depending upon the size of the goiter and the patient's desires.

THYROID DISORDERS

A mass in the front of the neck is usually due to a thyroid mass **(Table 40.1)**. It could be involving only one lobe of the thyroid or affecting both lobes. The mass can be small or big.

TABLE 40.1: Types of thyroid.

Benign	Neoplastic
Colloid goiter	Adenoma
Nodular goiter	Papillary carcinoma
Hashimoto's thyroiditis	Follicular carcinoma
Acute suppurative thyroiditis	Medullary carcinoma
Subacute thyroiditis	Lymphoma
Riedel struma	Hürthle cell carcinoma
Graves' disease	Anaplastic carcinoma
Myxedema	MEN syndrome
Cysts	

(MEN: multiple endocrine neoplasia)

All thyroid masses have certain characteristics. The mass moves with deglutition and is located directly in front of the neck and below the thyroid cartilage and is mostly slow-growing and painless in nature.

The mass should be palpated from the back of the neck as well as from the front of the neck. Assess the nodularity or mass for size, mobility, and number of masses **(Box 40.1)**. Assess the trachea for deviation. See if the mass lifts up and if the lower rim of the thyroid can be palpated. Look for any evidence of hyperthyroidism or hypothyroidism. Assess for any pressure symptoms and hoarseness of voice.

The two main tests for the thyroid are thyroid function tests and sonogram of the thyroid. FNA cytology of all nodules is done under sonogram guidance.

If the FNA is normal or colloid material, generally no surgery is needed unless the mass is big and the patient wants it done for cosmetic reasons. In these instances, lobectomy or subtotal lobectomy of the affected side is adequate **(Box 40.2)**.

BOX 40.1: Thyroid—tests.
- TSH level—high level indicates low activity of thyroid gland. Low level indicates well-functioning thyroid
- T3 and T4 levels—high levels indicate well-functioning gland and vice versa
- Sonogram—identifies the nodules, solid versus cystic
- Nuclear scan—identifies hot nodule, cold nodule
- FNA—obtains cellular material for cytology

(FNA: fine-needle aspiration; TSH: thyroid-stimulating hormone)

BOX 40.2: Thyroid—treatment.
- Medical treatment—for benign small, diffuse goiters, hyper- or hypothyroidism, post-thyroid surgery, small nodular goiters
- Use thyroid-stimulating hormone, T3, T4 as guidelines
- Thyroid supplements, Synthroid, levothyroxine
- Antithyroid medications—propylthiouracil, Tapazole (methimazole), iodine, propranolol
- Radioiodine ablation

A benign goiter can be treated with thyroid suppression and dietary advice. Iodine deficiency is endemic in many areas with resulting goiters. Iodine supplements are helpful in this situation. Surgery is done when a nodular goiter is large. At times, they form a large cyst—they can be aspirated with a fine needle and observed for recurrence.

If the sonogram shows no well-defined masses, but the patient has a diffuse goiter, then thyroid function tests are used to place them on thyroid suppression therapy. If the thyroid-stimulating hormone (TSH) is high, thyroid supplements are increased and vice versa.

CANCERS OF THYROID

Treatment of thyroid malignancies is best planned with a multidisciplinary team consisting of surgeon, radiation oncologist, medical oncologist, and endocrinologist, along with other members of medical caregivers.

Risk assessment is done based on specific histology, lymph node status, metastatic status, and the patient's medical condition. 80% of all thyroid cancers are papillary cancers which fortunately are slow-growing cancers with a better prognosis.

If the FNA is abnormal, suspicious of malignancy, or shows cellular material, then surgery is done to remove the mass. All malignant nodules or suspected malignancies are best treated with total thyroidectomy to avoid further surgical procedures and to facilitate adjuvant therapy.

Papillary carcinomas have better prognosis; therefore, some surgeons advocate total thyroidectomy on the same side and near-total thyroidectomy on the contralateral side. Follicular carcinoma and Hürthle cell carcinoma are best treated by total thyroidectomy. However, surgery is avoided in anaplastic cancer of thyroid gland, which is treated with radiation and chemotherapy since surgery is dangerous and prognosis is poor. If medullary carcinoma is the diagnosis, one should do total thyroidectomy with bilateral radical neck dissection and evaluate the patient for multiple endocrine neoplasia (MEN) syndrome.

Radioactive iodine (RAI) is a useful tool to manage remnants of cancer cells or spread to lymph nodes or distant sites. Patients will need lifelong thyroid supplements and follow-up with endocrinologist after thyroid surgery or radioablation therapy. The status of lymph nodes is assessed with the use of ultrasound, computed tomography (CT) scan of neck, and positron emission tomography (PET) scans. When needed, ultrasound-guided FNA cytology is used. If there is evidence of spread to lymph nodes, partial or complete neck dissections are done for best cancer clearance.

Graves' disease is initially treated with antithyroid medications. If still uncontrolled, the choice is between radioiodine ablation and near-total thyroidectomy. If the thyroid function tests show evidence of hyperthyroidism, the patient is placed on antithyroid medications such as thiouracils or methimazole. The dosage is adjusted based on follow-up thyroid function tests.

Hashimoto's thyroiditis is an autoimmune disorder and can present with varying findings. Often, the diagnosis is made from the pathology report after a lobectomy for nodule. Subacute thyroiditis is another autoimmune disorder. If diagnosed correctly by FNA, they can be placed on steroids or anti-inflammatory agents. Riedel struma or thyroiditis causes compression on the trachea and esophagus since it has a hard cicatrix with fibrous tissue causing progressive constriction. Isthmusectomy is recommended to relieve compression on the trachea.

> **BOX 40.3:** Thyroid—surgery.
>
> - Lobectomy or partial thyroidectomy for benign conditions, cysts, colloid goiter, unilateral nodular goiter, cosmetic concerns
> - Total or near-total thyroidectomy for cellular or atypical fine needle aspiration, suspected or confirmed malignancies, Graves' disease, and substernal thyroid (no surgery for anaplastic carcinoma)
> - Division of isthmus for Riedel struma
> - *Identification and preservation of recurrent laryngeal nerve:* Recurrent laryngeal nerve is a white glistening nerve fiber in tracheoesophageal groove, running along the back of trachea toward the larynx. Do not use electrocautery or harmonic scalpel in this part of dissection. Stay flush on the thyroid capsule and lift the thyroid lobe upward and toward the midline during the dissection. Another option is to leave a small amount of thyroid tissue at the tracheoesophageal groove and dissect through the thyroid gland if it is being done for a benign condition. Some surgeons use a nerve stimulator, but the author never uses them. Do not touch or manipulate the nerve in any fashion. Just identify and stay away from it
> - *Identification and preservation of parathyroid glands:* Usually there are four parathyroid glands, two in upper poles and two in lower poles. They are brownish-yellow in color and different from fat-yellow. They are more well defined than fat. There is a cluster of blood vessels next to it. Keep the dissection flush with the thyroid capsule, and slowly but steadily tie off or use bipolar to take down the small veins and arteries entering the thyroid capsule. The parathyroids will separate off at the upper and lower poles
> - *Getting good hemostasis:* Keep the dissection meticulous and slow. Raise the flap under the platysma on top of pretracheal fascia. Suture ligate large veins in situ at the upper and lower ends of field. Get into the plane flush with thyroid capsule. Ligate larger vessels in continuity on the patient side and then divide toward the specimen side with bipolar. Divide strap muscles if exposure is difficult. Pack the wound for a short time if there is welling of blood and then go back with suitable retractors and nontoothed forceps. Use hemoclips when tying is difficult. Place a closed suction drain for 24 hours if there is oozing

Substernal goiters can be operated on from the neck most of the time since the blood supply is from the neck, and the thyroid can be delivered from the superior mediastinum to the neck. However, one should be prepared for a median sternotomy for difficult or large retrosternal thyroid masses **(Box 40.3)**.

Newer modalities of thyroid surgery are attempted that include remote access surgery to avoid a scar in the front of neck. The approaches tried are from axilla, chest, or oral cavity. Newer instruments, flexible tools with robotics, and precise energy devices along with nerve monitoring intraoperatively have made these possible. However, open neck surgery is still the standard of care.

Postoperatively after thyroid surgery, one should look out for:
- Thyroid storm—patient is tachycardic, dehydrated, has fever, and goes into a shock-like state. Treat with hydration, steroids, Inderal or propranolol, and antithyroid medications.
- Hypothyroidism—treat with thyroid supplements on a long-term basis.
- Hypoparathyroidism—treat with calcium and vitamin D.
- Bleeding and hematoma—evacuate the hematoma and obtain good hemostasis.
- Recurrent laryngeal nerve injuries—watch for hoarseness of voice and dyspnea—may need airway protection, tracheostomy, ear, nose, and throat (ENT) consultation, and voice training.

KEY POINTS

A mass in the front of the neck is usually related to the thyroid. Thyroid function tests and sonogram are the two main tests. FNA of the mass is obtained. If any type of abnormality is noted on the FNA, plan for a total thyroidectomy.

CHAPTER 41

Thyroglossal Duct Cyst

INTRODUCTION

This is a congenital lesion related to the development of the thyroid gland. The thyroid gland originates at the base of the tongue at the foramen cecum and then migrates down to the normal location in front of the neck. In the process, it can leave behind a track that goes through the hyoid bone and can develop into a cyst along the track. The classic sign is the mass moves with protrusion of the tongue. The most important thing to remember is not to incise and drain it thinking it is an abscess.

EVALUATION AND MANAGEMENT

Thyroglossal duct cyst is located above the thyroid cartilage, near the midline but slightly off to one side, as a spherical soft small mass under the chin. This is a remnant of the track from the foramen cecum in the base of the tongue, where the thyroid gland originated in the first place.

Diagnosis

For the most part, diagnosis is by clinical examination and high degree of suspicion. The classic location, rounded cystic appearance, being slightly off the midline, and the movement of the cyst with protrusion of the tongue are unique features. Thyroid masses move with deglutition, whereas the thyroglossal cyst moves with protrusion of the tongue. Ultrasound examination of the cyst will be useful. There is no need for any other thyroid-related tests.

Caution

Do not incise or aspirate the cyst. It needs proper surgery in the operating room, with excision of the whole cyst and its tract in continuity along with a segment of the hyoid bone. One should not aspirate or do an incision and drainage of the thyroglossal cyst since it will lead to a persistently draining fistulous tract.

Treatment

Surgery for thyroglossal duct cyst is known as Sistrunk's operation. A transverse incision is made at a level just above the mass, and flaps are raised in the pretracheal plane. The entire mass is dissected from the lower end and slowly dissected upward when a clear well-defined track can be noticed. The track is dissected up to the hyoid bone, where a segment of the bone is cut along the track. Then the track is traced up to the base of the tongue, where it is securely ligated and divided. Failure to do the complete excision of the cyst and entire track will lead to recurrence.

While open surgery has been the time-honored treatment, newer modalities are being tried.

Robotic surgery has been utilized to make precise dissection and smaller incisions with faster recovery.

Another development has been injection of sclerosing agents under ultrasound guidance into the cyst, which results in fibrosis and collapse of the cyst, thus avoiding need for any surgery. The reported results show lesser complications and lesser chance for recurrence, with excellent results. The sclerosing agents used are ethanol or another agent called OK-432, which is deactivated and modified strain of *Streptococcus pyogenes*. This creates an immune response resulting in fibrosis and obliteration of the cyst. Large cysts may need repeat injections.

KEY POINTS

A complete formal excision as described above is needed. Other than the physical examination and high index of suspicion, no specific test is required to confirm the diagnosis. Ultrasound-guided injection of sclerosing agents appear to be effective, thus avoiding the need for surgery.

Mass on Side of Neck: Lymph Nodes

INTRODUCTION

Enlarged lymph nodes can be nonspecific but usually are related to some type of infection. However, it can also be a primary malignancy of lymph nodes such as lymphoma or a secondary spread of malignancy from another part of the body. Fine needle aspiration (FNA) of the lymph node is the best course of investigation if malignancy is suspected. If necessary, a complete excision of a lymph node is done for further tissue diagnosis and special stains. They may need additional tests such as complete blood count, liver chemistries, sonogram, or a computed tomography (CT) scan for further evaluations.

DIAGNOSIS

A mass on the side of the neck is most commonly an enlarged lymph node. Other causes depending upon the site could be due to an enlarged submaxillary salivary gland, parotid mass, carotid body tumor, or pharyngeal diverticulum.

Most of the enlarged lymph nodes are of infectious origin **(Fig. 42.1)**. They could be due to bacterial, viral, or fungal in nature. Some of them are acute suppurative, such as cat scratch disease, while others are chronic caseating, such as tuberculosis.

However, the enlarged node could be related to a malignant process. It can be a primary lymph node pathology such as lymphoma or a secondary metastasis from carcinoma elsewhere. The primary cancer can be in the head and neck region itself, such as nasopharynx, oropharynx, and hypopharynx, or it could be in thyroid, lung, visceral organs such as gastrointestinal (GI) tract, or ovary, breast, and skin lesions.

Multiple enlarged nodes that are discrete, rounded, and slightly mobile on both sides of the neck along with generalized lymphadenopathy are suggestive of primary lymph nodular malignancy such as Hodgkin's disease, lymphosarcoma, lymphocytic leukemia, and

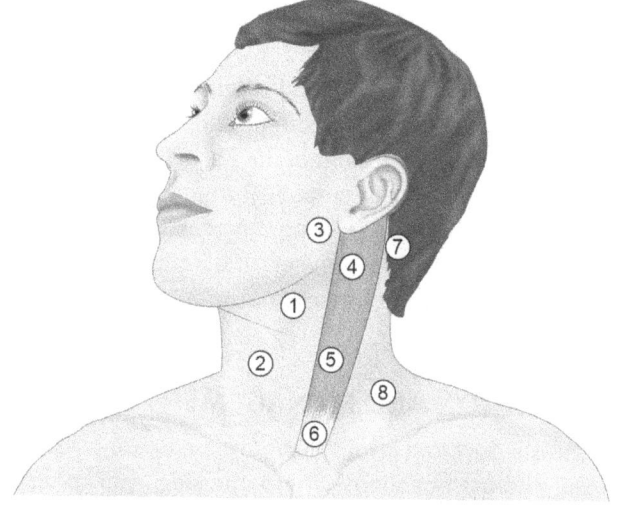

1. Submental—Submandibular salivary gland or lymph node.
2. Front of neck—Thyroid, thyroglossal cyst
3. Subauricular angle of mandible— Parotid gland
4. Upper jugular ⎤
5. Mid jugular ⎥ Lymph node
6. Supraclavicular ⎬ Lymph node
7. Occipital ⎥
8. Posterior ⎦

Fig. 42.1: Mass on the side of neck—lymph nodes.

myeloproliferative disorders **(Table 42.1)**. These patients may have associated hepatosplenomegaly. Staging of the disease is needed to define whether they are supradiaphragmatic, infradiaphragmatic, or generalized in deciding radiation and/or chemotherapy.

One or two small, rounded nodes in the occipital region with no other nodes are probably a scalp infection. Small isolated submaxillary lymph node is probably related to oral cavity infections, dental problems, or gingivitis. Sometimes, they are mistaken for submandibular sialadenitis.

A very hard, immobile glandular mass on one side of the neck with no other generalized lymphadenopathy is suggestive of a metastatic spread with primary in the head

TABLE 42.1: Enlarged lymph nodes.	
Benign	**Primary malignancy**
Bacterial infections	Lymphomas
Viral infections	Hodgkin's disease
Spirochetes	Lymphosarcoma
Cat scratch disease	Leukemias
Tuberculosis	Histiocytoma
Fungal infections	*Secondary malignancy spread*
HIV/AIDS	From head and neck, ovaries, breast, GI tract, lungs, thyroid, testes, skin
Autoimmune disorders	
Infectious mononucleosis	

(AIDS: acquired immunodeficiency syndrome; GI: gastrointestinal; HIV: human immunodeficiency virus)

BOX 42.1: Enlarged lymph nodes—treatment.
- Find the underlying cause and treat the same
- Look for a primary cancer thoroughly
- FNA, sonogram, chest X-ray, and CT scan are helpful
- Complete excision biopsy with special stains and markers as needed
- Medical therapy directed to the causative agent
- Chemotherapy and radiation for lymphomas and primary lymph node malignancies
- Wide radical resection, composite resections for curable secondary malignancies

(CT: computed tomography; FNA: fine needle aspiration)

and neck region. This could be in the oral cavity, tongue, palate, nasopharynx, hypopharynx, skin, scalp, or thyroid. These patients may need radical neck dissections along with radical resection of the primary site.

Virchow's nodes refer to a hard supraclavicular metastatic lymph node. This could be a spread from the abdominal cavity or any of the visceral organs, ovary or testicle, lung or breast.

There is an entity of occult primary to be kept in mind. In these cases, a metastatic lymph node is confirmed in the neck by FNA or core biopsy. However, a primary cannot be found. The hidden areas in the head and neck region could be in the larynx, hypopharynx, nasopharynx, or in the sinuses. Melanomas are known to shrink, or they had excision done in the past. They will require a CT scan, magnetic resonance imaging (MRI) of the head and neck, laryngoscopy, and upper GI endoscopy.

A good history and physical examination can lead to a possible diagnosis. FNA of the lymph node can yield valuable information. At times, a complete excision of one lymph node is requested for good tissue diagnosis and marker studies.

A sonogram of the mass is recommended when the mass is suspected to be other than an enlarged lymph node. Depending upon the diagnosis, an additional workup such as a CT scan of the chest or abdomen is ordered.

Further treatment depends upon the exact diagnosis. Infections are treated with antibiotics. Lymphomas need chemotherapy. Malignancies may need radical resections depending on the stage of the disease **(Box 42.1)**. Supplemental radiation or chemotherapy is added.

Surgical Points

Lymph node biopsy: Mark the area in sitting position and in supine position before anesthesia is administered. Once the patient is positioned appropriately, the site may shift and may not be well palpable afterward. A patient's neck will need to be extended or tilted to get best exposure of the site. Recheck the position of the lymph node after positioning the patient before prepping and draping. The lymph nodes feel superficial very often. However, they are deep to the neck fascia and will require dissection deeper than expected. Be aware of nerves, arteries, and veins in the vicinity. The best strategy is to get into the false capsule overlying the lymph node and dissect flush with the lymph node instead of dissecting in the tissues around the lymph node. If the lymph node feels adherent or hard to enucleate in full, take out only a visible part of the lymph node for purpose of biopsy, and do not persist with bigger dissection. The patient may have malignancy that needs a different strategy for treatment.

KEY POINTS

Most masses on the side of the neck are due to enlarged lymph nodes. Most enlarged lymph nodes are due to some type of infection. FNA is a good starting point.

SECTION 6

Breast

43. Mass in the Breast
44. Pain in the Breast
45. Bleeding or Discharge from the Nipple
46. Gynecomastia
47. Abnormal Mammogram

CHAPTER 43: Mass in the Breast

INTRODUCTION

Breast cancer is a common form of cancer and has a good chance of cure if diagnosed and treated early. A screening mammography is the best available screening test to detect nonpalpable breast pathologies. Unfortunately, it is neither available nor performed widely in many parts of the world, where the first sign of concern arises only when a lesion has become palpable. Because of fear, taboo, or ignorance, they seek medical advice late, by which time the chances of cure are less. Moreover, due to cost concerns, delinquencies in keeping follow-up visits, and advanced stage of the disease, most of them end up with modified radical mastectomy, with very few breast conservation procedures with adjuvant radiation and chemotherapy **(Fig. 43.1)**.

EVALUATION AND MANAGEMENT

Every mass in the breast, whether noted by the patient or by the physician, must be followed to conclusion because of the possibility of carcinoma **(Box 43.1)**.

A rounded, firm, mobile, and smooth mass in a young person is probably a fibroadenoma. A hard, irregular mass with restricted mobility or tethering of skin in a middle-aged or older person is probably a carcinoma. A vague thickening on a recent-onset vague mass with pain in childbearing age is probably a fibrocystic disease. These three entities make up the majority of breast lumps.

A complete history-taking and physical examination along with an evaluation of risk factors for carcinoma are important.

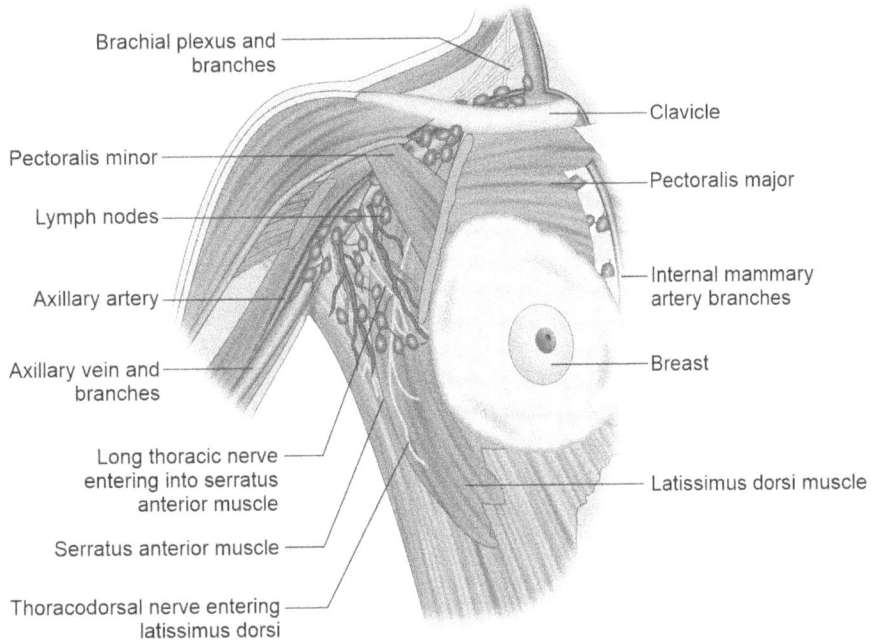

Fig. 43.1: Modified radical mastectomy/axillary node dissection.

> **BOX 43.1:** Mass in the breast.
>
> - Fibroadenoma—young patient, well defined, smooth, mobile, firm in consistency
> - Carcinoma—older patient, irregular and hard, restricted mobility, tethering of skin
> - Fibrocystic disease—young patient, ill-defined area of thickening or cyst formation, mild tenderness, multiple small nodularities
> - Bedside needle aspiration—if cystic fluid (clear, turbid, greenish, or brownish) is aspirated and mass disappears, the patient can be reexamined in 6 weeks, assuming that this is benign process. If no fluid is aspirated, it can be used for fine-needle aspiration purpose

> **BOX 43.2:** Mass in the breast—tests.
>
> - Sonogram—useful to know if the mass is solid or cystic, finds deep-seated masses, clarifies physical examination findings, assists in obtaining FNA, core needle biopsies, and in removing the benign masses with mammotome
> - Mammogram—useful to know about deep-seated abnormalities, finding microcalcifications, clarifies physical examination findings, evaluates opposite breast, best screening test for general public, assists in stereotactic biopsies, and in removal of benign masses using mammotome
> - MRI of breast—useful to further evaluate a mass when other tests are indeterminate, assists in MRI-guided biopsies

(FNA: fine-needle aspiration; MRI: magnetic resonance imaging)

> **BOX 43.3:** Carcinoma of breast—diagnosis.
>
> - High index of suspicion from physical examination, sonogram, or mammogram
> - Fine-needle aspiration—sonogram-guided or mammogram-guided
> - Tru-cut needle or mammotome needle core biopsies—sonogram-guided or mammogram-guided
> - Wire needle localization and excision biopsy
> - Incision biopsy or excision biopsy at surgery

Mammograms are done as screening tests or upon detection of a lump. The three conditions described above have distinct appearances in a mammogram **(Box 43.2)**. Fibroadenoma looks as a rounded, well-marginated, solid mass. Carcinoma appears as an irregular, speculated solid mass **(Box 43.3)**. Fibrocystic disease shows vague densities with ill-defined edges.

Incidental findings in mammograms are microcalcifications and deep-seated, nonpalpable lesions.

The next test is usually an ultrasound of the breast. This can differentiate between a solid and a cystic lesion. Cystic lesions can be aspirated with or without ultrasound guidance. The fluid can be sent for cytology even though the yield is very minimal. If the mass disappears after aspiration of fluid, it can be followed clinically as a benign fibrocystic disease.

A solid palpable mass can be biopsied with a needle, either as core needle Tru-cut biopsy or by doing a fine-needle aspiration (FNA). If the lesion is suggestive of a benign fibroadenoma by clinical and mammographic impressions and confirmed to be so with FNA or core needle biopsy, a complete local excision can still be done if the patient so desires in order to avoid continued follow-up and uncertainty in the minds of patients. This will be the final step in their treatment.

Currently, many of the suspected breast lesions are diagnosed with a core needle biopsy or FNA cytology. Biopsies of nonpalpable lesions can be done with a special mammotome table setup and devices or by ultrasound-guided techniques. Many such lesions are nonpalpable to start with but detected under routine screening mammogram or other imaging modalities. Hence, it becomes necessary to leave a marker at the biopsy site, to facilitate definitive surgery for margin clear wide excision later. Some such methods are:

- *Mage seed:* A radiologist places a magnetic seed at the site of biopsy the day before. It is followed at the time of excisional procedure.
- Faxitron and Hologic are companies that have products for localization and high resolution imaging.
- Ultrasound-guided localization at the site of hematoma or at the site of MammoStar marker.
- Needle localization of the marked site just before surgery, with the patient transported to the operating room (OR) with the needle in place, and it is followed by surgery.

Any suspicion of carcinoma with either FNA or core needle biopsy must be followed by planned cancer surgery. The ideal option today is to do a wide local excision or margin clear lumpectomy along with sentinel node biopsy. If the sentinel nodes are positive, then a complete axillary lymph node dissection is done. This is to be followed by radiation, chemotherapy, or hormonal therapy based on specific details **(Boxes 43.4 to 43.7)**.

An alternate option is to do a modified radical mastectomy **(Box 43.5)**. In many developing countries, a modified radical mastectomy is the preferred treatment for all breast cancers, since patients may not return for follow-up radiation and chemotherapy due to cost concerns as well as logistical concerns.

Patients will need radiation and/or chemotherapy after surgery for cancer, depending upon a variety of factors. If a patient did not have a mastectomy, radiation therapy is recommended to the remaining breast since it is cancer prone and can have recurrence. Intensity-modulated

BOX 43.4: Carcinoma of breast—treatment.

- *Surgery:* Modified radical mastectomy, wide excision lumpectomy with sentinel node biopsy of axilla, followed by full axillary node dissection, if necessary, total mastectomy
- *Chemotherapy:* If the nodes are positive, if the primary is >1 cm in size, if hormone assays are negative, for inflammatory carcinoma. Neoadjuvant preoperative therapy
- *Radiation therapy:* If no mastectomy is done, to treat remaining breast after breast conservation surgery, for stage 3 and 4 carcinoma
- *Hormone therapy:* If hormone assays warrant the same using antiestrogens (tamoxifen, aromatase inhibitors)
- *Targeted therapy with human epidermal growth factor receptor 2 inhibitors (trastuzumab, pertuzumab)*

BOX 43.5: Modified radical mastectomy—surgical techniques.

- Avoid raising very thin skin flaps—they may necrose and wound edges may become ischemic
- En bloc removal of breast and axillary contents through the same incision is done
- Secure ligation or suture ligation of branches of the internal mammary artery before they retract under the muscle or into the chest wall
- Finding and preserving the thoracodorsal nerve and long thoracic nerve in the axilla. Long thoracic nerve runs along the chest wall and supplies serratus anterior and thoracodorsal nerve runs on the back wall of axilla over the latissimus dorsi muscle which it supplies
- Avoid injury to axillary vein, axillary artery, and brachial plexus. Find the axillary vein and keep the dissection inferior to it all the time

BOX 43.6: Sentinel node biopsy.

- Inject Technetium-99m in the periareolar area in the nuclear lab before bringing the patient to the operating room
- Inject methylene blue or Lymphazurin in the periareolar area and give a 5-minute soft breast massage
- Open the axilla with a small transverse incision
- Use "navigator" probe to look for "hot" uptake area
- Look for blue color node
- Sentinel node is one that is hot, blue, hot and blue and that is visible and palpable
- Remove the sentinel node, check on the back table for hot uptake, and recheck the wound for loss of the hot area that was previously noted
- Send the node for frozen section—if it is grossly positive, convert the surgery to a complete node dissection at the same sitting
- *Warning:* Totally absent hot or blue uptake can be due to massive metastasis in the axilla and blocked lymphatic. Do a complete axillary node dissection in these instances

BOX 43.7: Hormonal therapy.

- Estrogen and progesterone assays—ER and PR positives can be given hormone therapy—about 70% of breast cancers are positive—drugs—tamoxifen, Arimidex (anastrozole), Femara (letrozole), Aromasin (exemestane)
- HER2 (human epidermal growth factor receptor 2)—20% of breast cancers have HER2 positive (over expression). These patients can benefit from Herceptin (trastuzumab) therapy. HER2 negative has better prognosis and does not need this monoclonal antibody therapy
- Triple negatives are those who are ER and PR negative and HER2 positive. They must be given chemotherapy since they have a worse prognosis. Immunotherapy is an option then.

(ER: estrogen; HER2: human epidermal growth factor receptor 2; PR: progesterone)

radiation therapy and proton beam therapy are being used for better precision and less side effects. If the breast cancer is >1 cm in size or if it has spread to any of the lymph nodes, then chemotherapy is advised to avoid systemic recurrence.

Hormone assays on the tumor are done to know if they are estrogen and progesterone sensitive or not. If they are negative, chemotherapy is advised. If they are positive, one may elect to give antiestrogen medication such as tamoxifen.

The most common form of breast cancer is scirrhous type, which is an invasive cancer of the breast presenting as a hard irregular mass with tethering to the subcutaneous tissue and restricted mobility. Lobular carcinoma arising from the lobules has a tendency for bilaterality; hence, both breasts should be checked. Inflammatory carcinoma has extensive subcutaneous lymphatic spread of the cancer and the whole breast turns into cancer without a distinct palpable mass. It is a rapidly spreading severe form of cancer. Paget's disease of the nipple presents as an ulcerated eczematous-type lesion of the nipple but has an underlying ductal malignancy.

Phyllodes tumor is a malignant transformation of a very large fibroadenoma, arising from mesenchymal cells.

Similar to other cancers, breast cancer also requires a team approach for better coordination between all the caregivers. Some surgeons have become specialized in breast surgery, and some radiologists have become specialized in breast services to include investigations and different types of image-guided needle biopsies. Participation by medical oncologists and radiation oncologists is equally important.

KEY POINTS

All breast masses should be fully evaluated and treated. Fibroadenoma, fibrocystic disease, and cancers are the three main items to be considered. A mammogram, sonogram, and a needle biopsy or FNA will help in making final decisions.

CHAPTER 44

Pain in the Breast

INTRODUCTION

Most patients think that pain is a symptom of breast cancer; however, most breast cancers are painless to begin with. Pain is benign and self-limiting in pubertal changes. Menstrual cycles can have episodes of pain or discomfort. Fibrocystic disease is a common cause of pain. Acute mastitis, breast abscess, and trauma are the other causes of pain.

DIAGNOSIS AND TREATMENT

Pain in the breast, also known as mastodynia or mastalgia, is usually a benign condition, even though patients think of cancer. The causes could be fibrocystic disease, pubertal changes, trauma, mastitis, or breast abscess. Other causes of pain in the breast include hormonal changes during menstrual periods, pregnancy, or due to medications such as hormones and contraceptives. Trauma to the breast or to the chest wall muscles or ribs can present as breast pain. Rare occurrences of inflammatory cancer of breast can present with redness and pain over the breast.

Patients with fibrocystic disease complain of vague discomfort in the breast, with worsening symptoms during menstrual periods. A physical examination shows vague thickening with ill-defined edges. Sometimes, well-defined cysts are noted. A mammogram and sonogram show vague densities with or without cyst formations. Conservative treatment is best advised for these patients. Avoidance of cola drinks, caffeine, and chocolates is helpful. Medications such as danazol, evening primrose oil, bromocriptine, and tamoxifen are prescribed. However, these are contraindicated if the mastalgia is due to pregnancy. Analgesics and non-steroidal pain medications are useful.

Infections can gain access through the nipple areola and milk ducts. In acute mastitis, there is redness and inflammation of the skin and subcutaneous tissue. Once an abscess is formed, a mass is formed associated with tenderness. A sonogram confirms a cystic cavity, and aspiration of pus is confirmatory. Antibiotics are started. The abscess must be drained once confirmed.

KEY POINTS

Consider fibrocystic disease or breast infection as the first diagnosis when someone complains of pain in the breast.

CHAPTER 45

Bleeding or Discharge from the Nipple

INTRODUCTION

Discharge from the nipple can be normal physiology or it can be abnormal and require medical attention. Factors that raise the suspicion of malignancy include blood drainage, unilateral drainage, associated mass, or abnormal mammogram with drainage. Duct papilloma or duct carcinoma is a concern if there is blood coming out of the nipple.

DIAGNOSIS AND TREATMENT

It is alarming and annoying to the patient to notice abnormal discharge from the nipple. Many patients may have physiologic discharge. They involve both nipples. Obviously, pregnancy and lactation are normal physiology.

Bilateral yellow to green discharges can be caused by estrogens, tranquilizers, or sexual stimulation. They are nonspecific and small in quantity. These patients need only reassurance and observation. Infections such as breast abscess or mastitis can cause drainage from the nipple. These patients will be benefited from antibiotic therapy.

Drainage of dark fluid, brownish fluid, and at times greenish fluid is usually related to fibrocystic disease. A cyst is in direct continuity with a major milk duct and it finds its way out through the milk duct. The patient is concerned with hygiene and her undergarments getting soiled. If the problem is persistent, a subareolar milk duct excision is done along the offending milk duct. A tiny lacrimal probe can be advanced through the nipple opening as a guide for excising the quadrant.

Sometimes it is red blood, but more often it is just brownish fluid mistaken as blood by the patient. The causes of red blood could be duct papilloma or duct carcinoma. A mammogram and sonogram may not show any abnormality. One could send a smear of the drainage fluid for cytology. A ductogram by injecting radiopaque material into the draining focus can be done. However, the best option is to do surgery—segmental excision of the subareolar milk duct is done after identifying the involved milk duct by probing. An adequate deep excision of the problem-bearing area is done. If a carcinoma is identified, it is treated as any other breast cancer, per protocol.

KEY POINTS

Excision of subareolar milk duct is the best treatment for persistent drainage of blood or brownish drainage from milk duct.

CHAPTER 46

Gynecomastia

INTRODUCTION

Enlargement of the male breast is gynecomastia. It can be benign and physiologic during puberty and old age. However, it can also be pathologic during medical conditions and diseases. More serious is male breast cancer, which can appear as gynecomastia. All gynecomastia cases need proper physical examination and evaluation.

DIAGNOSIS AND TREATMENT

It is an enlargement of the male breast. It can be uncomfortable and painful at times when it is rubbing against clothes. Patients are also concerned about the cosmetic appearance and psychological effects. They seek surgical help because of these issues.

This is a benign condition, often self-limiting. Etiology could be due to intake of certain medications such as antitestosterone drugs used for an enlarged prostate (Avodart® and Proscar®), cardiac medicines such as digoxin, antacids such as Pepcid®, or use of cannabis. Pubertal changes as well as old age can cause prominent male breast. Liver diseases, testicular abnormalities, and hormone anomalies are other causes.

It is important to examine the patient to make sure that one is not missing male breast cancer. In carcinoma of the male breast, there is a very hard mass attached to the skin or areola with restricted mobility. There could be nipple retraction, dimpling of the skin, or nipple drainage. Spread to the axillary nodes is common, presenting as enlarged lymph nodes in the axilla. This is different from Paget's disease of the nipple, which is also a form of breast carcinoma. In Paget's disease, there is an eczematous-type ulceration of the nipple. Biopsy in the form of incisional or Tru-cut will be diagnostic. Many physicians order a mammogram or an ultrasound for further workup. However, they do not add much to the clinical information.

Treatment is directed to the underlying cause. Surgical excision of the gynecomastia by doing a subareolar subcutaneous mastectomy is very effective. Male breast cancer is treated by modified radical mastectomy. Male breast cancers carry a worse prognosis than female breast cancers because of delayed diagnosis, earlier spread to lymph nodes, and less sensitivity to hormone manipulations. Hence, they need aggressive treatment with multimodality therapy in addition to radical surgery.

KEY POINTS

Gynecomastia is usually a benign condition. However, one must always rule out a male breast carcinoma.

CHAPTER 47

Abnormal Mammogram

INTRODUCTION

A mammogram is the best available screening test to detect nonpalpable breast lesions. It is a routine wellness procedure as part of regular checkups. It can detect nonpalpable masses and microcalcifications, which can be a harbinger of cancer. It also helps to evaluate the contralateral breast when cancer has been diagnosed on one side. The question arises as to what to do when an abnormal spot has been detected on the mammogram—how to biopsy these areas, which one can be observed, and which one to treat. It can also bring in a certain amount of controversy regarding how far to go on an asymptomatic lesion.

DIAGNOSIS AND TREATMENT

It is not uncommon for patients to walk into a surgeon's office or clinic with a mammogram that has been done elsewhere. It is probably done as a routine screening procedure or done to evaluate some suspected abnormality. These patients are tensed, since someone in the healthcare system has already advised them to go to a surgeon, and the patient interprets it as a serious matter.

Hence, it is important to be calm and polite with them. A proper history taking and physical examination are done to know if there are any palpable masses. The surgeon must carefully review the mammogram and the report. All surgeons who deal with breast lesions should be able to read and interpret a mammogram independently, while at the same time reviewing the report initiated by the radiologist. The advent of digital mammography and assistance with artificial intelligence have made more accuracy in the test results. Both breasts should be evaluated by physical examination as well as by a mammogram for comparison.

Abnormalities in the mammogram include mass lesions, microcalcifications, densities, and parenchymal distortions. The main goal of doing screening mammogram is to identify cancers at an early stage, for better cure rate and better chance for breast conservation surgery. Not all abnormalities are cancers; however, all abnormalities should be confirmed of their diagnosis, with biopsies and with follow-up.

At times, there are microcalcifications. If they are very coarse, they are probably benign. Inside of an old fibroadenoma, there can be one or two blotches of calcium. Calcium can get deposited on the walls of arteries following lines of these blood vessels. All of these can be observed.

If they are clustered, small, and powdery, there could be cancer in this area. One should do a stereotactic core needle biopsy to rule out malignancy in these areas. If the core needle biopsy is anything but completely normal, then a complete local excision of the abnormal area is done with the help of wire needle localization.

An alternate option is to do a mammogram-guided wire needle location and wide excision of the area bearing microcalcification as first-line surgery. Further management for carcinoma is done if such diagnosis is confirmed.

Radiologists with special interest have become interventional breast radiologists and perform needle biopsies and fine aspiration cytology, to the extent that only malignant conditions that require further management are referred to the surgeon.

Other times, one may see nonpalpable mass lesions. Features of the mass can indicate whether they are malignant or not. Cancerous masses have spiculated margins, jagged edges, and irregular borders. Benign lesions such as fibroadenoma have well-defined rounded, clear-cut edges. In the case of fibrocystic disease, one may see clear rounded cystic shadows or just thickened dense parenchyma. They must be biopsied similarly and treated accordingly.

There are situations when the mammogram is too dense to read or has multiple indeterminate spots.

Asymmetry of parenchymal density between two sides is a matter of concern. A magnetic resonance imaging (MRI) of the breast as well as a sonogram can be done for further evaluation. MRI-guided needle biopsy is an option.

Irrespective of the course of action, all these patients should be followed up with yearly mammograms and physical examinations.

KEY POINTS

An abnormal mammogram should be carefully evaluated. Any questionable or suspicious areas should be biopsied either by sonogram-guided, stereotactic mammogram-guided using Mammotome or by excision biopsy. A mammogram is the best screening test available to detect nonpalpable cancers early on.

SECTION 7

Groin Conditions

48. Mass in the Groin
49. Mass in the Scrotum
50. Urological Problems in General Surgery
51. Hernia

CHAPTER 48

Mass in the Groin

INTRODUCTION

Usual masses in the groin are hernias, either inguinal or femoral. At times, they are enlarged lymph nodes. Other soft-tissue pathologies are rarely considered. A physical examination and history can guide in making the diagnosis. A reducible mass that disappears early in the morning is a common history for a hernia. A nonreducible tender mass that suddenly appeared with severe pain is probably a strangulated hernia. A long-standing large inguinoscrotal mass is probably a chronically incarcerated hernia.

DIAGNOSIS AND TREATMENT

Patients sometimes state that they noticed a lump in the groin area. It could be a hernia, an enlarged lymph node, or rarely other pathologies.

A hernia could be inguinal or femoral. A hernia is a protrusion of the internal viscera through a defect in the abdominal wall, often through a natural area of weakness. When it comes out through the inguinal canal, it is an inguinal hernia. When it comes out through the femoral canal, it is a femoral hernia.

A physical examination can differentiate the conditions. Lymph nodes are small, rounded, nonreducible, often multiple in numbers, often bilateral, and have distinct margins around each of the nodes. They are located slightly lateral in the uppermost thigh area, just below the inguinal ligament.

An inguinal hernia is a softer, reducible, larger mass with an expansile impulse on coughing, presenting as a large single globular or slightly elongated mass just below or at the inguinal ligament on the medial side of the groin. A finger can be placed into the inguinal canal through the scrotal skin by invaginating it, and an impulse of hernia can be felt on the fingertip as the patient coughs.

A femoral hernia is felt as a rounded mass located just below the inguinal ligament on the medial side of groin, medial to the femoral artery, and more common in women. Inguinal hernia is still a more common form of hernia in both men and women. When the hernia is incarcerated, they can be tender and nonreducible.

A large hydrocele can be mistaken for an inguinoscrotal hernia. In the hydrocele, one can get above the mass and can pinch the spermatic cord by itself above the mass, and the testicle cannot be separately palpated below the mass. There is fluid fluctuation and positive transillumination. In the case of an inguinoscrotal hernia, it is difficult to feel the spermatic cord separately above the mass, but the testicle can be palpated separately.

If the clinical diagnosis is uncertain, a computed tomography (CT) scan of the area is the best confirmatory test. The defect and hernia protrusion can be clearly seen. In the case of enlarged lymph nodes, evaluation of other nodes such as iliac nodes and para-aortic nodes, as well as the status of the liver and spleen, can be made.

A hernia needs surgical repair. The basic principles are to dissect the hernia, address the contents by reducing it, address the sac by removing the sac or in certain cases pushing it back, and then repair the defect. Many different techniques are involved for the different hernias, by open method or by laparoscopic method or by robotic-assisted method. Mesh reinforcement has become the standard for most hernia repairs.

Hernia in children and young adults is congenital in origin, where the peritoneal lining that descends with the testicle does not close off at the deep inguinal ring. In these cases, a herniotomy is adequate without repair of the floor of the inguinal canal, where the hernia sac is separated at the external ring, and the proximal end going into the abdominal cavity is closed off or tied off.

In Bassini repair, the shelving edge of the inguinal ligament is sutured to transversalis aponeurosis. In McVay repair, the pectinate ligament is sutured to transversalis aponeurosis. In Shouldice repair, the layers are sutured with running Prolene. In Lichtenstein tension-free repair, the floor is sutured with a mesh in place. In the laparoscopic method, the sac is separated and pushed back, and a large piece of mesh is placed against the defect and tacked in place. In the robotic assistance, the procedure is the same as with laparoscopic repair, but fine dissection and suturing are done more precisely. In laparoscopic and robotic procedures, a space is created in the preperitoneal space with a spacemaker first. In transabdominal preperitoneal (TAPP) repair, space is created between the peritoneum and the abdominal wall, after entering into peritoneal cavity and a mesh is placed against the defect. Bilateral hernia repair can be done with the same approach. In total extraperitoneal (TEP) repair, the extraperitoneal space is directly approached on one side, after creating a space between abdominal wall and peritoneum using a balloon dissector. Both have become the preferred approach compared to the intraperitoneal approach. In these types of repairs, the incisions are smaller, with less postoperative pain resulting in earlier ambulation and return to work. However, the high costs, availability of necessary instruments, and familiarity of setup are drawbacks. In the long-term, the differences are not significant. Hence, most countries still use the open repair for the vast majority of hernia repairs.

Lymph nodes can be further evaluated by fine-needle aspiration (FNA) or biopsy. Further treatment depends upon the exact diagnosis.

KEY POINTS

A physical examination is of utmost importance to differentiate between an enlarged lymph node and a hernia. If there is doubt, obtain a CT scan.

CHAPTER 49

Mass in the Scrotum

INTRODUCTION

A mass in the scrotum can be sudden in onset and painful. One has to consider torsion of the testicle or acute epididymo-orchitis in these cases. A long-standing, slowly progressive, and painless swelling can be a hydrocele or an inguinoscrotal hernia. A sudden painful inflammation of the skin of the scrotum associated with fever can be Fournier's gangrene. A carcinoma of the testes has to be kept in mind in all scrotal swellings.

DIAGNOSIS AND TREATMENT

A mass presenting in the scrotum can be arising from the testes, tunica vaginalis, or a hernia. A mass of the testes can be epididymo-orchitis or testicular tumor.

Fluid around the testes accumulating inside the tunica vaginalis is a hydrocele. An inguinoscrotal hernia can be mistaken for a hydrocele and vice versa.

A physical examination is helpful to differentiate them. In the case of hydrocele, one can feel the fluctuation by holding the whole scrotum between two hands. The testes cannot be felt separately from the fluctuant mass since it is located inside the fluid-filled sac. Transillumination can show a clear fluid. It is possible to pinch the cord structures above the mass. Hydrocele is treated by surgical excision or eversion of the sac.

In the case of a hernia, one cannot get above the mass since it is coming from inside the abdomen. However, the testes can be felt separately in the scrotum and below the mass in most instances. Expansile impulse on coughing and extension of the mass to a level above the inguinal canal is also diagnostic. A hernia requires surgical repair as described in the previous Chapter 48.

A testicular mass is a solid, separately palpable mass inside the scrotum. This can be a testicular cancer. A testicular biopsy is needed for diagnosis. Treatment will require radical surgery and possible para-aortic lymph node dissection followed by chemotherapy, depending upon the exact pathology.

When the testes or the epididymis is enlarged and tender, it is an inflammatory process such as epididymo-orchitis. A very tender testicle of sudden onset can be due to acute torsion of the testicle. At times, it may be difficult to differentiate between an acute epididymo-orchitis and acute torsion of the testes. A sonogram with arterial Doppler can evaluate the status of the testes and blood supply. Sometimes, emergency exploration of the scrotum is necessary if the diagnosis is uncertain. Epididymo-orchitis is treated with antibiotics; torsion is treated by surgery with detorsion and orchiopexy. Orchiectomy will be needed if it has become totally ischemic.

Varicocele is engorged and tortuous veins in the scrotum. While most of them are asymptomatic and have no consequence, one must rule out renal tumors or compression of the testicular veins. They can cause fertility impairment. If they are symptomatic, excision of the varicocele can be done.

Trauma can cause swelling of the scrotum. This can be seen after surgery for hernia. Injuries of the scrotum can occur following blunt trauma.

Lymphedema of the scrotum can present as swelling. Filariasis is common in tropical countries. It can also be due to lymphatic obstructions from other reasons.

Hematocele is accumulation of blood in the scrotal sac. It is usually due to trauma, surgery, or testicular cancers.

Spermatocele is a localized collection of fluid in the spermatic cord, appearing as a small, rounded mass just above the testicle, with mild fluctuation.

Fournier's gangrene is a surgical emergency. The patient develops acute necrotizing infection of the skin and subcutaneous tissue of the scrotum, with rapid spread up to the groin level above and up to the perianal level below. There is associated bacteremia, sepsis, fever, and tachycardia. They go into septic shock, and necrosis can extend further along the tissue planes. Broad-spectrum intravenous (IV) antibiotics are started, and wide incision drainage with debridement of all necrotic tissue is done. The patient may need two or three sittings of radical debridement surgery. Usually, the tunica vaginalis is spared and testes remain viable. The wound is left open and will slowly heal by secondary intension.

KEY POINTS

A careful physical examination can differentiate between a hernia, hydrocele, and testicular mass. An ultrasound with arterial Doppler is helpful. Appropriate surgical correction will be needed.

CHAPTER 50

Urological Problems in General Surgery

INTRODUCTION

Urology is a well-recognized specialty now. However, many parts of the world are still underserved and general surgeons handle most of the common urological problems. Even otherwise, general surgeons should be familiar with ordinary urological problems, particularly those that can be done as outpatient procedures.

CIRCUMCISION

Circumcision is a commonly done procedure in children for hygienic and religious reasons. It can be done under general anesthesia or local anesthesia. During circumcision in children, it is easy to cause injury to the penis if due care is not taken. An adequate rim of the inner skin is kept to suture it to the trimmed-off portion of the outer skin. It is important to secure good hemostasis before closing the edges. An interrupted absorbable suture is placed for closing. Circumcision has medical benefits, such as reduction of sexually transmitted infections, carcinoma of penis, urinary tract infections, and chance of paraphimosis. It increases hygienic care also.

PARAPHIMOSIS

In paraphimosis, the prepuce of the penis gets pulled back for some reason and does not go back. It forms a very tight ring with a tourniquet type resulting in severe pain, inflammation, and edema. As time goes by, it becomes more and more difficult to reduce it. If diagnosed early, using manual efforts and mild lubricants, it can be reduced. If diagnosed late, one will have to inject local anesthesia and divide it carefully and reduce it. Afterward, a dorsal split or circumcision can be done.

SEXUALLY TRANSMITTED DISEASES

Patients with purulent discharge from the urethra, stricture of urethra, warts and granulomas, herpes, syphilis, and human immunodeficiency virus/acquired immunodeficiency syndrome (HIV/AIDS) come to the physician for treatment. Appropriate antibiotic therapy, education on safe sex, and use of condoms are the first-line treatments.

VASECTOMY

Vasectomy is a frequently done procedure for family planning purposes. The procedure, consent, and potential failure of the surgery should be discussed in detail with the patient. It can be done as an office procedure under local anesthesia. The vas deferens is brought tight against the scrotal skin, keeping it pinched against the index and thumb of one hand. The other hand is used to inject the local anesthetic and make a small 1 cm sized incision directly over the vas deferens. Using a sharp, large curved needle, the vas is stabilized on top of the needle, and careful incisions are made over the spermatic fascia to dissect out the glistening whip-like vas deferens for a length of 2 cm. It is ligated at two ends, and about 1 cm length of the vas is excised. The specimen is sent to histology for tissue confirmation. The patient is advised to continue the precautions against pregnancy, such as use of condoms, intrauterine device (IUD), or birth control pills for about 6 weeks, to ensure that already stored sperms are eliminated from the body. In addition, the author advises them to obtain a semen analysis to ensure that sperms are absent in the semen before stopping those antifertility measures.

URINARY TRACT INFECTIONS

Patients frequently complain of fever, chills, burning pain on micturition, flank pain, and suprapubic pain. There is tenderness over the renal angle and over the flank area. Simple urinalysis can show pus cells, RBCs, or bacteria. Often, this is adequate to start them on antibiotic therapy. Urine cultures can be obtained for specific therapy. Investigations can be undertaken to detect any causative factors, and attention is directed toward them.

RETENTION OF URINE

The most common reason for retention of urine would be an enlarged prostate. Other causes include stricture of urethra, trauma, rupture of urethra, medications, and neurological injuries. Efforts are made to insert a Foley catheter and find the underlying causative factor. Sometimes, an insertion of a Foley catheter may be difficult. Lubricating the urethra and catheter liberally, using a smaller-sized semi-stiff red rubber coudé tip catheter with a tapering tip, use of dilators with caution, and use of filiforms with a follow-up catheter are various tips. Sometimes, one may have to do a suprapubic aspiration or a suprapubic cystostomy to overcome the emergency situation to avoid rupture of the urinary bladder. The patient can then be referred to a qualified urologist for further management.

Other problems such as hydrocele, hernia, Fournier's gangrene, torsion of testes, and varicocele have been addressed elsewhere.

KEY POINTS

General surgeons should be able to recognize and treat ordinary urological problems.

CHAPTER 51

Hernia

INTRODUCTION

The word hernia for a layman adult implies inguinal hernia. However, by definition, a hernia is simply translocation of an organ or part of an organ from its natural habitat to another location. Thus, theoretically, any organ can herniate. Most hernias need surgical correction since it is a mechanical problem.

DIAGNOSIS AND TREATMENT

A hernia is defined as when one body part protrudes out of its natural cavity or space to another space or cavity. Thus, a hernia can be external or internal. Depending upon the location, it is named inguinal, femoral, umbilical, epigastric, obturator, Spigelian, or lumbar. It can be reducible or nonreducible, incarcerated, or strangulated. A ventral hernia or incisional hernia is often related to prior abdominal surgery when the fascia layer has separated, leaving a defect under the skin.

An internal hernia can be the cause of intestinal obstruction or gangrene of the intestines. It can be caused by one loop of bowel herniating under another. It can herniate through a mesenteric defect following prior surgery, into the lesser sac, or into a mesenteric cavity in the pelvis. When a patient complains of severe abdominal pain with scant corroborating clinical findings, consider an internal hernia as a possible diagnosis. A hiatal hernia is herniation through the esophageal orifice, which can be a sliding hernia or a paraesophageal hernia.

Once diagnosed, all hernias should be evaluated for surgical repair. This is a mechanical problem, and medications will not correct the hernia (**Box 51.1**).

In plain language, when patients talk about hernia, they are referring to an external hernia, most commonly an inguinal hernia or incisional hernia.

> **BOX 51.1:** Inguinal hernia.
>
> - *Herniotomy:* For newborns, children, and young adults. The sac is identified, opened, and neck is ligated or sutured. No floor repair is needed
> - *Herniorrhaphy:* For adults and older individuals. The sac is identified, the contents are reduced, the neck of sac is sutured, or the ligated or entire sac is reduced back into the abdominal cavity, floor is repaired and reinforced with a mesh. Open surgery or laparoscopic approach or robotic assistance is done

INGUINAL HERNIA IN CHILDREN

As the testes migrate from the renal area to the scrotum, the peritoneal lining around it is supposed to close off at or before the deep inguinal ring, leaving only a covering around the testes itself as tunica vaginalis. Sometimes, this lining can continue to be patent for varying distances into the inguinal canal or all the way around the testes, thus causing the congenital hernia. There is no weakness of the abdominal wall in these instances. Hence, during the surgical repair, the key step is to identify the sac, open it to confirm the internal opening, and close it off from the peritoneal cavity. It is not necessary to dissect out the sac for its full length. The end toward the testes can be left open to prevent hydrocele formation. If the sac is wide and is difficult to separate entirely, a purse-string suture can be placed at the mouth of the opening from the peritoneal cavity, leaving the rest of the sac in situ. In children and young adults, this procedure known as "herniotomy" is adequate surgery. There is no need to do any repair of the floor of the inguinal canal.

INGUINAL HERNIA IN ADULTS

Many patients in this age group have an indirect hernia with a sac and weakness of the floor of the inguinal canal. The sac may have a congenital origin, but as time progresses, the floor also becomes weak. In these patients, it would be ideal to open the inguinal canal, tease out the sac from the cord structures, ligate the sac at its neck after making sure that the contents have been reduced back into the peritoneal cavity, and then repair the floor of the inguinal canal.

Despite various techniques, it has now become a standard practice to reinforce the floor of the inguinal canal with a patch of mesh.

Inguinal hernia can be classified as direct or indirect. In direct hernia, the floor of the inguinal canal has become so weak that it protrudes and bulges out. This occurs more in the elderly population. The hernia appears as rounded bulge on standing or coughing, closer to the pubic tuberosity toward the medial side. It reduces directly backward on compression. In the indirect hernia, the herniation traverses through the inguinal canal, following the spermatic cord, from the deep inguinal ring to the external inguinal ring and then down to the scrotum. Hence, the hernia has an oblique shape and reduces upward, laterally and then deep. It occurs more often in younger population. At times, a hernia can have both direct and indirect components together.

Different terminologies are given for different types of repair of the floor of the inguinal canal. Bassini repair is where the shelving edge of the inguinal ligament is sutured to transversalis fascia. McVay repair is where the pectinate ligament is sutured to transversalis fascia. Shouldice repair is where running sutures of Prolene® are made through all different layers of the floor. Lichtenstein repair is where a mesh is sutured to the edges with minimal tension. Marcy repair involves tightening the deep inguinal ring alone.

During the laparoscopic repair, the sac is pushed back into the peritoneal cavity after separating it out. The sac is also pushed back without opening it in direct inguinal hernia. Robotics has become more popular in repair of inguinal hernia as an extension of the laparoscopic approach. Different types of repairs are described, such as total extraperitoneal repair (TEP) or transabdominal preperitoneal repair (TAPP). The floor of the inguinal canal is reinforced with a mesh tacked in place.

INGUINAL HERNIA IN ELDERLY

Many patients in this age group have a patulous and weak floor of the inguinal canal, presenting as a direct inguinal hernia. The sac is often thick and, at times, incorporating the urinary bladder or colon in its wall with a wide mouth. The floor is the one to be repaired here, and it is best to push the whole sac back into the abdominal cavity, without dissecting it. The floor is then repaired with a mesh.

Ventral Hernia/Incisional Hernia

These are related to prior abdominal surgery where the deeper tissue has dehisced with healing of the skin and subcutaneous tissue. Obesity, smoking, infections, poor nutritional status, poor techniques, and poor immunological status are contributing factors. Elective repair can be done by the open technique, with placement of a mesh on the outside, or by the laparoscopic method, with placement of a mesh from the inside. Recurrent large ventral hernia may need component separation with reinforcement with a mesh.

KEY POINTS

All hernias should be evaluated for surgical repair since the underlying pathology is a mechanical defect.

SECTION 8

Vascular

52. Varicose Veins
53. Swelling of the Legs
54. Pain in the Legs
55. Numbness of the Legs or Hands
56. Gangrene of the Toes
57. Ulcerated Leg
58. Carotid Artery Surgery
59. Abdominal Aortic Aneurysm

CHAPTER 52

Varicose Veins

INTRODUCTION

Varicosities are engorged and tortuous veins. By colloquial understanding, it refers to prominent or visible veins in the lower extremity. They occur because of defective valves inside the veins, allowing gravity to make them bigger over a period of time. They can also occur because of obstruction to normal pathways, making them find alternative pathways. Very often, there is no specific cause. Treatment depends on the type and severity of varicosities and patient desires.

DIAGNOSIS AND TREATMENT

Engorged and tortuous veins cause concern both cosmetically and medically.

The etiology of varicose veins is unclear. Older age group, female gender, occupation that requires long periods of standing, pregnancy, obesity, and genetics are risk factors. Mostly, patients complain of engorged and tortuous visible veins under the skin. They may also feel aching sensation, swelling around the ankle, heaviness of the legs, and itching or burning sensation.

Many patients who come to the surgery clinic have a small cluster of prominent veins, sometimes visible as subcutaneous spider veins under the fair skin. These are concerns from a cosmetic point of view. They can be treated by injection of sclerotherapy agents or by surface lasers. Stab avulsion of the prominent veins is another option.

From a medical point of view, varicosities involving long saphenous system or short saphenous system are more significant. These are due to incompetence of major valves in the system, resulting in a backup of blood by gravity which causes an engorgement of the veins. Left alone, over a period of time, these veins can cause swelling of the calf, discoloration of the skin, chronic edema, and nonhealing ulcerations. Thrombosis of the veins can result in superficial thrombophlebitis, where palpable, tender, and red snake-like firm cords can be felt under the skin. Engorged veins can also bleed from minor trauma.

Initial treatment is with use of compressive stockings, lifestyle changes, and elevation of legs. Many noninvasive or minimally invasive techniques have been developed that give good results without the need for surgery with long incisions. Endovenous thermal ablation using laser or radiofrequency energy can be done under local anesthesia with sonogram guidance. Foam sclerotherapy aims to close the veins with a sclerosing agent. Medical adhesive and sealant are used in VenaSeal system. Mechanical agitation of the vein with injection of sclerosant is used in ClariVein system.

Surgery is often required to correct these varicose veins. Prior to surgery, it is recommended to do an ultrasound of the deep veins in the leg to know if there is deep vein thrombosis (DVT) or not. If there is DVT, surgery is avoided, and the patient is placed on anticoagulation. If there is no evidence of DVT, one can treat the varicose veins by surgery or ablation. Usually, it would involve stripping and multiple ligations of the long or short saphenous system.

Incompetent perforators in the leg can result in swelling, nonhealing ulcerations, and superficial varicosities. Subfacial ligation of the perforators by open surgery or video-assisted techniques can be done. Ultrasound-guided sclerotherapy has been used.

Secondary clusters of varicosities occur due to deep vein insufficiency. In these instances, the valves in the deep veins are defective, resulting in swelling of the legs, lymphedema, chronic dermatitis, and ulcerations. There is a great deal of pressure to excise these surface veins and stripping of the veins. However, such steps do not contribute to the control of the basic problem of deep vein insufficiency.

Varicosities can occur following obstructions of major vein pathways, such as portal hypertension or inferior vena cava obstruction. The prominence of such veins is due to veins finding alternative pathways. Efforts should be directed at reestablishing venous pathways such as portosystemic shunts or stent placement by the transjugular intrahepatic portosystemic shunt (TIPS) procedure.

KEY POINTS

Do an ultrasound of the deep veins to rule out DVT before undertaking surgical treatment or ablation of varicose veins.

CHAPTER 53

Swelling of the Legs

INTRODUCTION

Swelling of both legs can be due to a systemic problem resulting in edema. The cause could be cardiac, nutritional, or renal in origin. It can also be due to inferior vena cava obstruction. Unilateral swelling is due to deep vein insufficiency, deep vein thrombosis (DVT), or lymphedema. Sudden onset and painful swelling are due to DVT or infections. Most others are slowly progressive and painless. Treatment depends upon the exact cause.

DIAGNOSIS AND TREATMENT

Swelling of the legs can be unilateral or bilateral, chronic and long-standing, acute and short in duration, and painful or painless **(Box 53.1)**.

Bilateral swelling with pitting edema is usually related to generalized edema. This could be related to cardiac, renal, hepatic, nutritional, or intra-abdominal problems. They are treated with diuretics and investigated appropriately to find medical literature support for the root cause analysis.

Unilateral swelling could be due to iliac vein compression, lymphedema, DVT, or chronic venous stasis.

Painful swelling is due to infections such as cellulitis, ischemia of muscles, or DVT. DVT is treated with anticoagulants. Initially, a heparin drip is started and then converted to oral anticoagulants such as Coumadin® for a period of 6 months.

Recent-onset swelling is related to acute DVT, infections, or compartmental syndromes. Long-standing swellings are due to lymphedema or chronic venous stasis.

A physical examination and careful history will give a clue. A sonogram of the entire venous system will show any evidence of DVT or obstructions. A computed tomography (CT) scan of the abdomen and pelvis is useful to know if there are any pelvic tumors and will also give a good idea about iliac veins and inferior vena cava. A venogram is quite confirmatory of venous pathology.

Multiparous women have a combination of pelvic discomfort, chronic leg swelling, varicose veins, bladder symptoms, and chronic pelvic pain. It could be called pelvic congestion syndrome and is difficult to treat satisfactorily.

Chronic lymphedema and chronic venous stasis are difficult to be corrected by surgery, even though they get operated for excision of the secondary varicosities with no real improvement. It is important to avoid dry skin that can cause scratching, resulting in skin ulcerations and secondary infections. The skin is kept moist with moisturizing creams. The legs are kept elevated above the heart level. Application of compression bandages or use of lymphopress to keep the tissues soft is helpful. Surgical procedures attempted include lymphovenous anastomosis, excision of subcutaneous tissue and skin grafting for elephantiasis, and deep vein valve transplants.

> **BOX 53.1:** Swelling of the legs.
>
> - Bilateral—cardiac failure, renal failure, nutritional, fluid overload, vena cava obstruction, liver disease (usually pitting edema)
> - Unilateral—deep vein thrombosis, lymphedema, chronic venous insufficiency (usually nonpitting)
> - Tests—sonogram of calf veins, leg veins, abdomen, CT scan of pelvis and abdomen, venogram, lymphangiogram
> - Treatment—address the primary cause of swelling. For chronic lymphedema and chronic venous insufficiency, avoid skin ulcerations and secondary infections

(CT: computed tomography)

KEY POINTS

Bilateral swelling is usually due to systemic causes, and unilateral swelling is due to local causes. Chronic swelling is usually due to chronic venous insufficiency or lymphedema.

CHAPTER 54

Pain in the Legs

INTRODUCTION

Pain in the legs can be arterial, venous, infectious, traumatic, or neurological in origin. A careful history taking and physical examination are the starting points, and evaluations for one or more of the above factors need to be made. Arterial pain is marked by intermittent claudication, which later on leads to rest pain. Venous pain is felt in the calf muscles when associated with deep vein thrombosis (DVT). Neurological pain is radiating sharp pain along the nerve fibers. Infections are associated with redness, swelling, and fever **(Table 54.1)**.

DIAGNOSIS AND TREATMENT

"My leg hurts."

Pain in the legs could be ischemic in origin, either acute or chronic. Other possibilities are trauma, venous occlusion, and neuromuscular causes.

The duration of pain, character of pain, the patient's own perception of the cause of pain, severity of pain, and factors that relieve the pain are significant in making an initial diagnosis. A physical examination with palpation of the pulses and arterial Doppler ultrasound will give further information.

Acute arterial ischemia could be embolic in origin, acute on chronic atherosclerosis, or related to compartment syndrome. A sudden onset of pain, paresthesia, paralysis, pulselessness, and pallor are the classic descriptions of acute embolus. The limb is cold to the touch, with tenderness of the muscles as the ischemia progresses. An arterial sonogram will show the level of occlusion of the artery with total absence of flow distally.

Treatment is to heparinize immediately and do an arteriogram to confirm the occlusive site. Evaluation for endovascular interventions or thrombolytic therapy can be done at the same time. Surgery, if necessary, must be done very soon to do an embolectomy and revascularization steps as needed.

Chronic pain in the legs due to slowly progressing arterial ischemia is usually due to atherosclerosis. Intermittent claudication is the classic description, where the pain gets worse on walking and gets relieved on resting. As the ischemia becomes worse, rest pain develops. The ankle-brachial index will show that the ratio is <50% in these cases. A computed tomography (CT) angiogram or magnetic resonance (MR) angiogram can be done to confirm the extent of the disease and level of occlusion. Evaluation is done for endovascular therapy or surgery, both of which can be done electively.

In cases of DVT, pain is felt mostly along the calf muscles and is associated with calf tenderness (Homan's sign). There may be associated swelling of the leg on the affected side. A sonogram is the most diagnostic test. If confirmed, the patient is anticoagulated. Usually, one starts them on heparin drip intravenously (IV) and then converts them to an oral anticoagulant such as Coumadin®. The anticoagulation is continued for 6 months to allow time for the clot to solidify, thrombose, or dissolve.

TABLE 54.1: Pain in the legs.

Acute arterial	Acute venous
• Sudden onset of pain	• Sudden onset of calf tenderness
• Pallor, paralysis	• Swelling of the leg
• Pulselessness, tenderness	• Palpable pulses
• Paresthesia, cool	• Homan's sign positive
Tests	*Tests*
• Doppler, sonogram	• Venous sonogram
• Angiogram	• Venogram
Treatment	*Treatment*
• Thrombolytic therapy	• Anticoagulation
• Surgical embolectomy	• Thrombolytic therapy
• Bypass procedures	• Vena cava filter placement
• Anticoagulation	• Watch for pulmonary emboli
• Watch for systemic emboli	

The possibility of trauma must be ruled out in all cases where there is pain of recent onset. There could be fractures, muscle tears, or ligamentous sprain. Compartment syndrome can be due to internal bleeding or sepsis. An X-ray of the limb is ordered along with a sonogram. Orthopedic consultation and decompressive fasciotomy may be needed.

Pain of neurological origin can be due to nerve compression or peripheral neuropathy. Pain is felt as shock-like electrical waves that travel along the distribution of the nerve. Peripheral neuropathy gives a "pins and needles" sensation at the distal extremities. Medical conditions such as gout, diabetes mellitus, different types of arthritis, chronic stress syndrome, and spinal cord problems can present as leg pain.

Deep-seated infections, lymphangitis, cellulitis, abscesses, and necrotizing fasciitis are other causes of pain. There are telltale evidences of infections with fever, leukocytosis, and tenderness.

KEY POINTS

A careful history taking and physical examination followed by arterial Doppler study will give an idea of the etiology. Further evaluation is performed using a CT angiogram or an MR angiogram.

CHAPTER 55: Numbness of the Legs or Hands

INTRODUCTION

Peripheral neuropathy can be a contributing factor for surgical problems such as onset of neuropathic ulcers, burns, joint problems, and nonhealing wounds. The etiology could be metabolic disorders such as diabetes mellitus, nerve compression disorders such as prolapsed intervertebral disk, post-traumatic nerve injuries, poisonings, or infectious conditions such as leprosy. Timely diagnosis and corrective measures can avoid permanent nerve damage **(Table 55.1)**.

DIAGNOSIS AND TREATMENT

Neuropathic problems can be acute or chronic. The most common chronic neuropathy is related to diabetes mellitus. Sensory nerve function is lost in the periphery leading to ulcerations, Charcot's joints, and ischemic changes. Numbness of distal parts of both lower extremities is noted. Other causes of peripheral neuropathy include spinal cord problems, medication side effects, primary nerve disorders, nutrition, toxic syndromes, and poisonings.

Acute sudden onset of neuropathy is due to trauma, previous surgery, injections, or infectious processes. Most of these patients may have motor function deficiency along with sensory deficiency. Foot drop and wrist drop can be elicited, and motor strength of various muscle groups can be elicited. Fracture of bones or dislocation of joints can compress the peripheral nerves. Supracondylar fracture is known to cause ulnar nerve compression.

Diagnosis and treatment of compartmental syndrome of the extremity need early action since it is an emergency. This can happen after trauma, acute infections, regional toxin inoculation from insect or snake bites, revascularization of an ischemic limb, and rapid rewarming and rehydration of the body. The limb feels very tight and tense, with pain and tenderness. Peripheral pulses can be feeble. The condition can lead to severe tissue damage despite viable circulation, at times resulting in amputation of the extremity. Immediate four-compartment long fasciotomy is done to decompress the muscles. The muscles will bulge out, and the wound will be covered with moist wet saline gauze initially. As the limb recovers from the edema, it slowly shrinks, and the open wounds can be closed secondarily or skin grafted. Sometimes, they can heal spontaneously.

Thoracic outlet syndrome, cervical rib, and scalenus muscle syndrome can cause brachial plexus compression or branches of it. Cervical spine disk disease, degenerative arthritis, and rheumatoid arthritis can cause varying nerve compressions. Similar conditions include carpal tunnel syndrome causing median nerve compression, ulnar nerve entrapment syndrome, radial nerve entrapment, and pronator syndrome, where median nerve compression occurs in the proximal forearm.

Tumors of the nerve such as neurofibroma, giant cell tumors, and a schwannoma can create nerve deficits. Metabolic syndromes, myxedema, pregnancy, fluid

TABLE 55.1: Peripheral neuropathy.

Medical conditions	Surgical conditions
Diabetes mellitus	Thoracic outlet syndrome
Renal failure	Cervical rib
Vitamin deficiency	Carpal tunnel syndrome
Poisoning lead, arsenic	Spinal cord injuries
Alcohol	Fracture, dislocations
Shingles	Compartment syndrome
Leprosy, syphilis	Meralgia paresthetica
Lupus, rheumatoid arthritis	Ulnar nerve entrapment
Guillain–Barré syndrome	Peroneal nerve entrapment
Cancer therapy	Electrical injuries
Medications	Iatrogenic injuries at surgery
Myxedema	Pronator syndrome
Fluid overload	Radial nerve entrapment

overload, compartment syndrome following blunt injury, and ischemic revascularization are conditions where nerve compression can occur, resulting in foot drop or wrist drop.

A sharp "pins and needles" sensation in the legs is experienced in certain neuropathic situations. Part of the reason could be ischemia of the nerve fibers. They can also present as a "glove and stocking" type of distribution of paresthesia.

Restless leg syndrome is a separate neurological disorder where the patient is unable to sleep due to a funny sensation in the feet while in bed at night. The problem is not evident in wakeful hours during the daytime.

KEY POINTS

Think of peripheral neuropathy when the patient complains of numbness of legs. The most common problem is diabetes mellitus.

CHAPTER 56

Gangrene of the Toes

INTRODUCTION

Gangrene is the terminal event of severe ischemia when the body part dies. In patients who have chronic peripheral vascular disease, the part slowly shrivels off, mummifies, and becomes black with no sensation or function. In cases of uncorrected acute ischemia, there is edema, necrosis, and wet gangrene. Wet gangrene can also occur following necrotizing soft-tissue infections, diabetic ulcers, or acute occlusion of all venous pathways resulting in venous gangrene.

DIAGNOSIS

Gangrene is the death of macroscopic tissue. Most patients with severe peripheral vascular disease end up with gangrene of the toes. Toes are the distal-most tissues of the body with the least vital functions.

Gangrenous toes can be single digit or multiple, presenting as a dark, shriveled, and mummified organ with no sensation or movements. It is essentially a dead organ. There is not enough blood supply to the distal foot to keep it viable anymore **(Box 56.1 and Fig. 56.1)**.

> **BOX 56.1:** Peripheral vascular disease.
>
> *Intermittent claudication*—cramping pain in calf muscles on walking relieved by rest
> *Rest pain*—worsening pain even at rest, awakens from sleep, relieved by dangling the foot over edge of bed
> - Onset of gangrene of toes, nonhealing ulcers
> - History of diabetes mellitus, hypertension, cardiac problems, carotid problems, smoking
> - Peripheral pulses become nonpalpable, hair loss, dry skin
> - Peripheral Doppler examination and ankle–brachial index
> - Duplex sonogram of peripheral vessels
> - CT angiogram or MR angiogram
> - Contrast digital angiogram

(CT: computed tomography; MR: magnetic resonance)

Patients give a history of peripheral vascular disease and progressively worsening symptoms. They start out with intermittent claudication and go on to develop rest pain. There is often a history of minor trauma to the toe or to the nail bed. There may be an associated neuropathy. Several of these patients have a history of smoking and a history of diabetes mellitus.

Intermittent claudication is a symptom complex where the patient experiences pain in the calf muscles upon walking or exercising. The pain eases off upon stopping the exercise and restarts again upon walking. This is because of diminished circulation to the calf muscles due to peripheral vascular disease. During exercise, there is demand for more blood flow and oxygen. In the absence of the same, the muscles feel the ischemic pain. The distance that the patient can walk without feeling pain is the claudication distance. As ischemia worsens, the claudication distance also falls. Eventually, it leads to pain at all the time. This phase is called rest pain. The patient often feels better by hanging the leg down.

The ankle–brachial (AB) ratio is calculated by comparing the blood pressure in the upper extremity with the lower extremity. Normally, it should be 1.00. When the AB ratio is 0.5, intermittent claudication is noted. When it falls to 0.25, rest pain sets in. Below this range, it leads to tissue loss and gangrene. Single-level blockage does not lead to gangrene because of effective collateral circulation.

The most common cause of gangrene of the toes is atherosclerotic disease. Plaque formation leads to occlusion and thrombosis of the artery. Once a vessel is occluded at one single spot, the occlusion usually extends up to the next major branch. Other causes of arterial disease are thromboangiitis obliterans (TAO), also known as Buerger's disease, Raynaud's disease, Takayasu's disease, scleroderma, and autoimmune disorders. It can happen following trauma to the extremity or postoperatively from complications resulting from aortoiliac/femoral arterial surgery. Popliteal

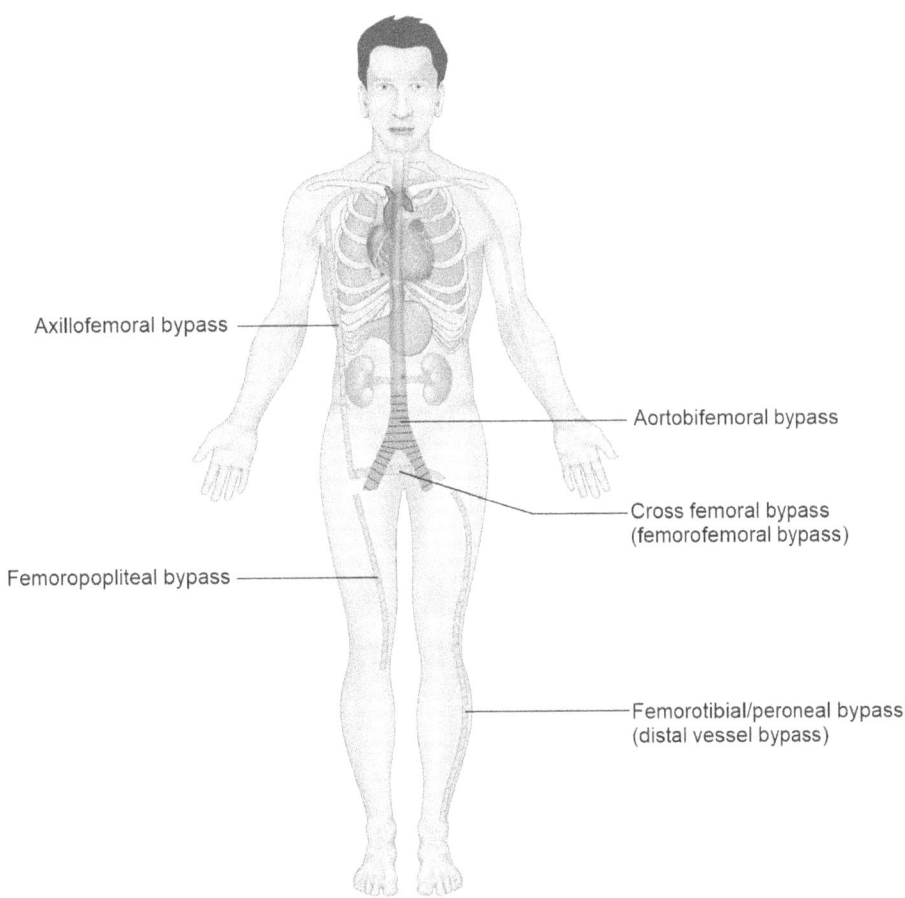

Fig. 56.1: Arterial bypass procedures for revascularization.

aneurysms can throw emboli to the distal vessels or can cause complete occlusion of all the arterial trees below the knee. Systemic embolization can occur from distant sources such as atrium or aorta. Dissection of intima of blood vessels resulting in occlusion can happen following cardiac catheterization or other endovascular interventions.

Dry gangrene of single toe can be allowed to shrivel instead of early amputation. The wound base will not heal properly until revascularization of the extremity has been established.

An arterial Doppler ultrasound and vascular examination will show occlusion of distal vessels. Usually, there are two areas of occlusion in the arterial tree before one develops gangrene of tissues. A computed tomography (CT) angiogram or magnetic resonance (MR) angiogram will confirm the levels of occlusion and extent of the disease. They are most commonly due to atherosclerosis.

Further management can be either by endovascular, open interventions, or hybrid procedures. It is necessary to revascularize the extremity; failure to do so will end up with amputation at the above-knee level or below-knee level.

Wet gangrene is a separate pathology related to necrosis of soft tissues, secondary to infections such as necrotizing fasciitis, diabetic ulcers, and soft-tissue infections. They can also be due to acute occlusion of arterial or venous blood flow. In these cases, there is swelling, pain, and patchy gangrenous changes of tissues. These patients require wide radical debridement, along with antibiotic therapy. Secondary corrective procedures or amputations at an appropriate level will be necessary.

Treatment

The primary focus is to reestablish vascularity to the extremity since vast majority of the cause of gangrene is atherosclerotic peripheral vascular disease related to occlusive plaques in the lumen. Endovascular interventions have taken a lead in recent years. These involve angioplasty and stent placements on localized segments of plaque formation. Completely occluded lumen can be recanalized using atherectomy and endarterectomy. Open surgical procedures involve a variety of bypass procedures to bring blood from above the area of occlusion to a level below the area of occlusion. Some of the options are shown in **Figure 56.1**. The bypass is done using a graft, which could be synthetic vascular grafts of various materials or could be an autogenous saphenous vein. Sometimes, hybrid procedures are done by combining endovascular and open procedures for maximum benefit.

KEY POINTS

Gangrene of the toes is the result of end-stage peripheral arterial occlusive disease, most likely due to atherosclerosis. Early investigation and revascularization may prevent amputation of the whole extremity.

CHAPTER 57

Ulcerated Leg

INTRODUCTION

Nonhealing ulcers in the leg could be due to arterial, venous, lymphatic, and neurological problems or certain infectious conditions. Some of them never heal, and the best one can hope is to avoid significant sepsis. Ulcers on the toes are usually ischemic in origin. Venous ulcers are usually on the medial side of the lower leg. In chronic lymphedema, the leg segment is firm, indurated, and the skin gets denuded for an extensive section between the knee and ankle. Neuropathic ulcers are on the sole of the foot.

DIAGNOSIS

Chronic ulcers and nonhealing wounds are common problems. A good history and physical examination can give clues to the etiology of these wounds.

It is possible that they may be arterial, venous, or neuropathic in origin. Infections of a different nature make it worse and problematic. Often, they start out as a small trauma such as an insect bite, careless nail paring, or a laceration. With added neuropathy and arterial or venous insufficiency, they deepen, and an infection burrows under the skin until a necrotizing soft-tissue infection develops. Once these infections are debrided, a large open wound is left behind. They may take a long time to heal or get worse over a period of time.

Patients with chronic venous insufficiency or lymphedema have hard, indurated soft tissues with unhealthy skin and subcutaneous tissue. Venous ulcers are usually located on the medial side of the lower leg, where maximal tissue induration occurs. Dryness of the skin causes itching. Scratching allows staph organisms to settle in, and sudden large areas of cellulitis or lymphangitis occur, resulting in denudation of large portions of the skin. These patients need intense local care, systemic antibiotics based on culture and sensitivity, and tight bandaging to reduce lymphedema.

Arterial wounds start as ischemic or gangrenous toes. These patients with chronic nonhealing wounds require improvement of arterial circulation.

Diabetes mellitus is the most common cause of neurological deficit. In places such as Africa or Asia, one should also think of leprosy or actinomycosis in the etiology.

TREATMENT

Wound care of chronic nonhealing wounds has become a specialty of surgery by itself because of the need for frequent monitoring and care. As a result, wound centers have sprung up attached to most hospitals. Most of their patients are related to chronic venous stasis, chronic lymphedema, and decubitus ulcers and are neuropathic in nature.

The principles of wound management are more or less the same irrespective of the causes. Adequate debridement of the wound and taking deep cultures are the first steps. The underlying cause needs correction. Antibiotics are administered as appropriate. Local wound care includes daily cleansing, covering the wound with moisturizing topical agents, and applying occlusive bandages. One such measure is the use of Unna boots, where tight bandaging is done with commercially available special elastic medicated plaster-like bandages that are changed once a week. There is a great tendency to use topical antibiotic creams; however, they are of minimal value and add to the cost of care. They may need secondary correction steps such as skin grafting or local amputations **(Box 57.1 and Fig. 57.1)**. Hyperbaric oxygen therapy has been used in the treatment of nonhealing wounds.

Surgical care of the underlying problem leading to an ulcerated leg depends on the etiology. Venous ulcers can be related to varicose veins, deep vein insufficiency, or incompetent perforators. Varicose veins can be treated by infrared or laser coagulation or by surgical stripping and multiple ligations. Deep vein insufficiency is due

> **BOX 57.1:** Wound care.
>
> - *Local care*—debride devitalized tissues, wound cultures, daily dressings, moisturizing agents, topical antibiotics, wound VAC application, ambulation
> - *Systemic care*—rectify arterial and venous insufficiencies, antibiotic therapy, nutritional support, care of neuropathy, rehabilitation and physiotherapy, hyperbaric oxygen, management of diabetes mellitus, hypertension, atherosclerosis, renal and pulmonary status
> - *Surgical care*—incision drainage of abscesses and debridement of necrotic tissue, amputations, skin grafts, arterial revascularization, venous surgery

> **BOX 57.2:** Snake bites.
>
> - Do not make incisions, apply tourniquet, or amputate the area of bite
> - Mark the area of bite, cleanse the wound, observe closely for vital signs, coagulopathy, neurological deficits, and allergic reactions, and watch for spread of the erythema and for compartment syndrome
> - Give antivenin therapy per protocol
> - Provide systemic support as warranted
> - Surgery—limited debridement of totally devitalized tissue and fasciotomy for compartment syndrome

(VAC: vacuum-assisted closure)

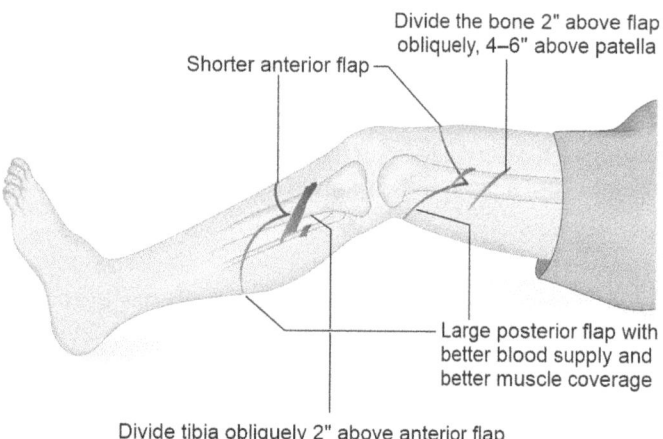

Fig. 57.1: Above-knee and below-knee amputations.

to incompetent deep valves. It is difficult to treat this effectively. Many of them have secondary clusters of venous engorgements, and the surgeon and patient are tempted to remove them by local excision. However, they do not correct the valvular incompetency of the deep venous system. Incompetent perforators can be treated by subfascial ligation of the perforators, either by laparoscopic-assisted way or by open surgery. All these patients need tight compression bandages for several days and elevation of the leg above the heart level.

Ulcers of arterial origin are mostly ischemic in nature and require appropriate revascularization of the extremity to ensure adequate blood supply to facilitate healing. Chronic lymphedema is also a difficult problem to solve by surgery. Several procedures, such as lymphovenous anastomosis and skin grafting after debulking the soft tissue, have been tried. No direct surgery is feasible for ulcers of neuropathic origin. They need proper preventive care, deep debridement, and possibly secondary corrective steps. Many of them result in amputation at an appropriate level.

Vacuum-assisted closure of a wound (wound VAC) has become a very useful tool in managing large open wounds anywhere in the body. Different companies have their products in the market. After proper debridement, wounds are covered by foam rubber with suction tubing on top and cellophane-type coverings over it. Closed suction is applied. The wounds slowly but steadily shrink in size. They are inspected once every 4 or 5 days, and new wound vacuum dressings are applied. The exact mechanism of action is still being debated. However, it reduces the need for daily wound dressings, soilage of dressings, and frequent nursing care, and the wound healing is rapid **(Box 57.2)**.

KEY POINTS

Chronic wounds in the lower extremities need patience and long-term care. The steps in the treatment procedure include correcting the etiological factors, adequate debridement, use of appropriate antibiotics, and local care of the wound.

CHAPTER 58

Carotid Artery Surgery

INTRODUCTION

Carotid stenosis is due to atherosclerotic plaque buildup at the carotid artery bifurcation between the external and the internal carotid arteries. The plaques encourage turbulence, platelet aggregation, and small clots to form and break off as distal emboli. The plaques can also break off or burst, resulting in sudden or slow narrowing of the lumen, and can eventually cause total occlusion. Carotid artery disease is one of the important causes of stroke and can be treated by early detection and surgery.

DIAGNOSIS

Carotid stenosis is a frequent cause of stroke. Stroke prevention should receive as much attention as prevention of heart attacks since it is one of the most common causes of death.

Atherosclerotic plaques buildup at the carotid bifurcation due to the shearing forces and turbulence of blood flow at this location. Once a plaque is formed, it slowly narrows the lumen and allows blood clots, platelet aggregates, and plaque materials to break off and become a source of emboli to the brain. Eventually, the artery can get completely occluded.

There can be many other reasons for stroke besides carotid artery stenosis. They include emboli arising from the heart related to atrial fibrillation, atrial myxoma, cardiomyopathy, trauma, intracranial bleeding, brain tumors, or intracranial arterial atherosclerosis. One will have to make a diligent effort to identify the cause of stroke while managing it at the same time.

TRANSIENT ISCHEMIC ATTACKS

Transient ischemic attacks (TIAs) have symptoms similar to a mini-stroke. The patient gives a history of transient weakness, paresthesia of one side of the body or one extremity with recovery after a while, transient blackout, syncopal episode, dizziness, slurring of speech, or transient blindness of one eye. The term amaurosis fugax is used to describe a set of visual changes related to embolic episodes in the retinal artery. This includes a sudden loss of vision in one eye or a curtain coming down over one eye suddenly and lifting up in the eye. The patient should be investigated for carotid artery disease whenever signs or symptoms of TIAs are suspected.

Another reason to initiate an investigation would be the presence of an audible carotid bruit on physical examination. A routine physical examination should include auscultation over the carotid artery to listen for a bruit.

A final reason to check the carotid arteries would be obvious and noticeable neurological deficits of any nature, whether it is hemiplegia, completed stroke, monoplegia, unsteady gait, or any central nervous system disorder.

TESTS

The first test is usually a duplex ultrasound of the carotid artery. One can evaluate the extent of narrowing, measure the flow velocities, and notice the status of arteries above and below the bifurcation. In certain instances, with a clear history and physical examination suggesting TIAs and if the duplex scan shows over 80% stenosis, then one can proceed for surgery of carotid endarterectomy without additional investigations.

If the sonogram is indeterminate, or if the patient has no clear symptoms of TIAs, then a second test is done. This can be either a magnetic resonance angiogram (MRA) or a computed tomography angiogram (CTA). These are imaging studies that show a better imaging picture of the carotid arteries as well as intracranial and extracranial circulation. Both tests can be done as an outpatient. A CTA needs a contrast injection.

If any ambiguity still lingers, then the final test would be a contrast angiogram done with digital subtraction. This is an invasive procedure that requires puncture of the femoral artery and injection of contrast material selectively into the carotid system.

If there is evidence of any neurological deficit or suspicion of past or present stroke, then a regular computed tomography (CT) scan or magnetic resonance imaging (MRI) of the brain is obtained immediately to know the current status of the brain. One must rule out intracranial bleeding.

TREATMENT

Evidence-based medicine and collective statistics show that a patient will be benefited by carotid endarterectomy if the stenosis is 80% or more in all patients or if the stenosis is 70% or more in patients with symptoms of TIAs. Without surgery, the risk of full stroke is 25% in 5 years, and with surgery, the risk of stroke is reduced to 1-5%.

The gold standard is to do a carotid endarterectomy. This involves a surgical procedure where an incision is made on the side of the neck; a carotid artery bifurcation is fully exposed with control of common carotid, internal carotid, and external carotid arteries; bifurcation is opened after anticoagulation; plaques that are builtup are removed; —the endarterectomy wound is closed with a patch to widen the site. The procedure has a risk of precipitating a stroke during the surgery in 1% instances or having partial neurological deficits without full stroke in 5% instances.

An alternative option of placing a carotid stent with angioplasty is being advanced as being a less invasive procedure. However, it also has various risks and potential to cause a stroke during the stent placement. With advancements in endovascular techniques, carotid artery stenting is gaining more popularity. To reduce distal embolization during the procedure, various modifications are introduced to trap and remove the debris during the procedure.

Another development is creation of stroke teams in acute care hospitals. If a new-onset stroke is diagnosed and treated within the first 4 hours of the onset of symptoms, the chance of full recovery from stroke is good. Emergency CT scan or MRI of the brain is done to make sure that there is no intracranial bleeding or tumors. Assuming there are no contraindications such as bleeding disorders, immediate administration of tissue plasminogen activator (tPA) can be injected as a form of thrombolytic therapy. The clots can be dissolved with a potential for recovery. Yet, another option is to consider intra-arterial selective embolectomy by the endovascular technique.

Once full stroke has set in, no immediate intervention is entertained. Physiotherapy, speech therapy, nutritional support, swallowing studies, decubitus care, occupational therapy, and rehabilitation are provided. After a period of 6 months, if the patient is otherwise stable, evaluation of the opposite carotid artery is done for prophylactic carotid endarterectomy or angioplasty as needed.

Surgical Techniques

Surgery of carotid endarterectomy can be done under cervical block or under general anesthesia. Some type of cerebral monitoring such as electroencephalography (EEG) is used during the procedure. The head is kept extended and turned to the opposite side. An incision is made along the anterior border of sternomastoid. Direct dissection of the common carotid artery is done by palpation. Entering inside the false lining around the artery, exposing the glistening arterial wall, will facilitate easier dissection than staying outside the fascia. The common facial vein must be divided and ligated to expose the bifurcation. Care is taken to avoid manipulating the bifurcation for fear of dislodging the plaque particles. The superior thyroid artery is the first branch of the external carotid artery, and it is controlled with a silk loop. Good exposure of internal and external carotid arteries is achieved. The hypoglossal nerve is identified and kept out of the way. If the dissection is kept flush with the arterial wall, one should not be seeing the vagus nerve or the glossopharyngeal nerve. Before clamping the vessels, heparin is given, and a small amount of lidocaine is injected at bifurcation. Most surgeons use a shunt to keep blood flowing from common carotid to internal carotid artery as soon as the artery is opened. Endarterectomy is done carefully to tapering edge at the ends. Most surgeons use a patch during closure to widen the area of endarterectomy. The shunt is removed before the last few throws of closure suture. After the procedure, the patient is checked for any neurological deficits.

At times, a patient presents with evidence of a totally occluded carotid artery on one side, with no neurological deficits. In these instances, one should not make any efforts to reopen the completely occluded carotid artery. The clots and occlusion can extend to a considerable distance intracranially, and the reopening steps can be dangerous. Moreover, the patient has good collateral circulation across the circle of Willis to maintain adequate perfusion of the entire brain. However, it would be prudent to check the contralateral carotid artery for stenosis. If there is over 70% narrowing of the contralateral carotid artery, then an appropriate intervention can be considered.

Another scenario is when a patient presents with a completed stroke on one side. The patient may be evaluated for carotid stenosis. If necessary, an intervention to correct any stenosis can be considered after a period of 6 months as a prophylaxis to protect the opposite side.

Medical management is considered for those who cannot have the above procedures or who do not agree for the interventions. It is also recommended for those who are at borderline risk without a clear indication for intervention. This includes diet, exercise, stress reduction, control of diabetes mellitus, hypertension, and use of aspirin or Plavix®.

KEY POINTS

Carotid stenosis is a common cause of stroke. Prophylactic carotid endarterectomy will be beneficial for the prevention of stroke in selected patients. A duplex sonogram and MRA are useful initial tests.

CHAPTER 59

Abdominal Aortic Aneurysm

INTRODUCTION

Abdominal aortic aneurysm (AAA) is asymptomatic until it ruptures, at which point it is a lethal situation. It would be ideal to detect the existence of AAA early on and treat them to prevent rupture. The wall of the abdominal aorta becomes weak, and it starts to dilate with a segment that balloons out. The most common cause is atherosclerotic disease. The best treatment is open repair of the AAA **(Fig. 59.1)** by replacing the diseased segment with a synthetic graft. Recent progress on endovascular repair, where a graft is placed inside of the aneurysm with a minimally invasive technique, has become very appealing as a simpler procedure.

ETIOLOGY

The exact etiology of an aneurysm is not understood. The most common cause is atherosclerosis. Infections of bacterial or syphilis nature can weaken the wall. Prior interventions with endovascular procedures or trauma can weaken the wall. Other risk factors are older age, smoking, male gender, high blood pressure, and family history. Certain

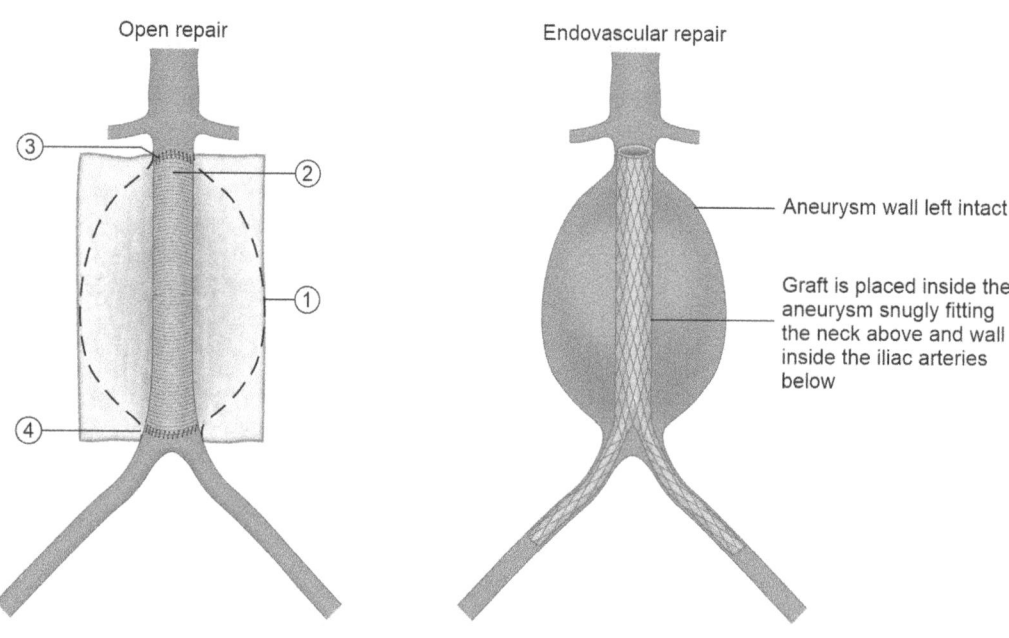

① Aneurysm wall in laid open
② A synthetic graft is sutured at upper and lower end of the aneurysm
③ Suture lines
④ Suture lines

Fig. 59.1: Repair of abdominal aortic aneurysm.

genetic conditions such as Marfan syndrome, Ehlers–Danlos syndrome, Loeys–Dietz syndrome, and Turner syndrome are known to cause aortic aneurysm.

DIAGNOSIS AND TREATMENT

An aneurysm is an expansion of the wall of an artery when the tubular arterial structure becomes ballooned out in one area. The wall becomes thin, and the ballooning becomes larger over a period of time, resulting in eventual rupture.

Aneurysms can occur in any part of the body. AAA is a problem that can be faced by a general surgeon from time to time. All aneurysms can become a life-threatening issue over time and require treatment upon diagnosis.

Abdominal aortic aneurysm remains asymptomatic until it ruptures. The diagnosis is at times made by a physical examination when a palpable pulsatile mass is felt in the upper abdomen. More often, they are noted as an incidental finding during an abdominal ultrasound, computed tomography (CT) scan, or magnetic resonance imaging (MRI) scan of the abdomen done for other reasons. Routine screening ultrasound examination of the abdomen is recommended once every 10 years for all above the age of 50 years for early detection.

Treatment of an AAA is by surgical correction. Elective repair can be planned after evaluating the size and nature of the aneurysm and its associated comorbidities. AAA is considered small at 4 cm, medium at 5 cm, and large at 6 cm, and an AAA of 5 cm or larger is considered an indication for surgery.

The time-tested method of surgery is by open surgical repair of the aneurysm. The aneurysmal segment of the artery is laid open and replaced by a synthetic graft. Associated stenosis or disease of iliac arteries can be overcome by using a bifurcated graft. Disease of the femoral arteries can be handled at the same time. Long-term results of a successful repair are good.

A saccular aneurysm (one wall is thinner than the other side) or a mycotic aneurysm (wall is infected) is likely to rupture even if they are small in size. Hence, they are also recommended to have surgery upon diagnosis.

An alternate option is endovascular aortic aneurysm repair (EVAR) by placement of an intra-aortic stent. In this procedure, a bifurcated graft is placed inside of the aneurysmal sac, snugly fitting it at the neck and at the iliac arteries, with the result the blood is now flowing through the newly placed graft, allowing the original wall to collapse over it. This is becoming more popular because it is a less invasive and quicker procedure. This is especially suitable for elderly individuals or those with various comorbidities.

The choice between open repair and endovascular repair is decided by several factors, such as the characteristics, size and length of the neck of the aneurysm, status of iliac arteries and distal arteries, age and comorbidities of the patient, surgeon experience and institutional amenities, cost concerns, and patient preferences. In general, younger patients are considered suitable for open repair, and older patients for endovascular repair. EVAR carries lower morbidity, postoperative mortality, and earlier ambulation, with reduced hospital stay. These patients need regular follow-up checks to rule out endoleaks and recurrence.

If an aneurysm is <5 cm in size, the patient must be followed up with a repeat ultrasound examination at 6-month intervals to make sure that it is not growing in size.

Symptoms of a ruptured aortic aneurysm must be kept in mind. There is extremely severe low back pain that is unrelenting and getting worse, followed by hypotension, sweating, abdominal distension, shock, and oliguria. It should be held in differential diagnosis in all unexplained cases of hypotension, shock, anemia, and back pain.

Confirmation can be quickly obtained at the bedside with a portable ultrasound, where the retroperitoneal hematoma and normal/dilated aorta can be noted. A CT scan is confirmatory; however, this can delay the treatment and increase the chance of mortality.

The best treatment is immediate surgery. The abdomen is opened by a long midline incision, the retroperitoneum is opened, and the aorta is quickly cross-clamped at the neck of the aneurysm. If this is difficult, then the aorta should be cross-clamped at the hiatal region. Simultaneously, the patient should be receiving a rapid infusion of intravenous (IV) fluids and blood, along with systemic support.

Several centers are now doing intra-aortic stent placement for ruptured aneurysms as the first-line treatment. They have proper staffing and the necessary equipment to facilitate the same.

KEY POINTS

An aortic aneurysm will be totally asymptomatic until it is ready to rupture. Elective repair of the aneurysm is recommended when it is 5 cm or more in size. This can be done by open surgery or by endovascular intra-aortic stent placement. Ruptured aneurysms have a high mortality and morbidity.

SECTION 9: Skin and Subcutaneous Tissue

60. Skin Lesions
61. Subcutaneous Lumps and Bumps
62. Ganglion Cyst
63. Skin and Subcutaneous Infections

CHAPTER 60

Skin Lesions

INTRODUCTION

Three common skin cancers are basal cell carcinoma, squamous cell carcinoma, and melanoma. It is important for the clinician to diagnose and treat them early when they are mostly curable. Melanoma is the most dangerous of them. Wide excision with skin grafting or flap closure is done for the primary lesion. Sentinel lymph node biopsy followed by selective radical node dissection is done for the lymph nodes. The cure rate goes down significantly once distant metastasis occurs.

DIAGNOSIS AND TREATMENT

Almost everyone has a skin lesion sometime or the other that causes concern. Most of them, however, are benign. The most common benign skin lesions are keratosis, pimples, and skin warts.

Keratosis appears as spots of thickened epidermis, usually in exposed areas to sunlight. The edges are sharp and well-defined with no other symptoms. They can be scraped, burned, or excised.

Pimples are clogged sweat glands usually on the face of young people during puberty. Frequent skin washings and topical application of Retin-A creams are useful. Avoiding secondary infections is necessary. The tendency to pick them with nails can cause bacterial infection.

Skin warts are pedunculated fibroepitheliomas that are benign in nature and cause irritation. Sometimes, they can be multiple and annoying. They can easily be burned or excised.

The three main types of skin cancers are basal cell carcinoma, squamous cell carcinoma, and melanoma.

Basal cell carcinomas are low-grade cancers appearing as a raised, ulcerated area with rolled edges and often with a brownish discoloration. It is the most common form of skin cancer. They commonly occur on the face, earlobes, and cheek. Wide local excision is curative in most cases. Radiation therapy also is effective.

Squamous cell cancers appear as scaly or ulcerated flat lesions, rarely with any pigmentation. They can arise on actinic skin damage, scars, and ulcers. They can occur in any part of the skin, but the face and upper and lower extremities are more prone. They tend to spread to regional lymph nodes. Wide radical excision is needed. Radiation therapy is an alternative when surgical excision is difficult.

Melanomas are the most dangerous variety, appearing as a pigmented lesion with spreading edges or ulcerated margins, sometimes with an itching sensation. They can spread to regional nodes as well as to distal organs via the bloodstream. Staging of melanoma depends upon the depth of invasion by Clark's level, Breslow's level, and regional node spread. Wide radical excision with sentinel lymph node dissection is done with possible regional radical lymph node dissection if necessary.

A less common form of skin cancer is Merkel cell carcinoma, which appears as a firm painless nodule on the exposed parts of the body. It is also an aggressive type of cancer that quickly spreads to regional lymph nodes. Wide radical excision, with radical dissection of regional lymph node, is recommended.

Evaluation of skin lesions, particularly for melanomas, is part of any routine physical examination. The patient should also bring any abnormal lesions to the doctor's attention. Any mole in the hands, feet, or face should be excised prophylactically. All pigmented skin lesions should be considered for biopsy to rule out malignancy. Patients are advised to avoid prolonged exposure to sunlight, apply sunscreen, and wear appropriate clothing when outside.

KEY POINTS

The three main skin cancers are basal cell carcinoma, squamous cell carcinoma, and melanoma. All efforts must be made to diagnose and treat them aggressively and early on.

CHAPTER 61

Subcutaneous Lumps and Bumps

INTRODUCTION

A bunch of outpatient surgeries or office surgeries comprise excision of "lumps and bumps." Many of them can be excised under local anesthesia, and fortunately, most are benign. They comprise sebaceous cysts, lipomas, synovial cysts or bursae, neurofibromas, and dermoid cysts. Lymph nodes, metastatic malignant nodules, and inflammatory nodules can also present as subcutaneous masses. A careful search for primary is made in these instances.

DIAGNOSIS AND TREATMENT

Patients present with various lumps and bumps and want to get rid of them. Fortunately, most of them are benign in nature. They can be sebaceous cysts, lipomas, neurofibromas, synovial cysts, or osteomas.

A sebaceous cyst is a collection of sebum or oily thickened putty-like material, collected internally from a clogged sweat gland. It can be present on the face, scalp, chest wall, or anywhere under the skin. Usually, a small punctum can be seen and felt when moving the skin over the mass. The skin over the mass is tight, stretched, and adherent at the punctum. It can get infected and present as an abscess or it can rupture, exuding a foul-smelling, cheesy necrotic material. It can be excised under local anesthesia by making an elliptical incision around the punctum.

A lipoma is a tumor of fatty tissue, benign in nature. The mass appears as a soft, mildly fluctuant deep subcutaneous lump with the overlying skin being completely mobile and free. The mass can be pushed slightly from side-to-side, showing no adherence to the tissue. They can be single or multiple, small or big. They can be excised under local anesthesia. The skin and subcutaneous tissue are incised when a plane over the mass can be found. Once dissection is kept on this false plane, the entire mass can be enucleated.

Neurofibromas can be multiple and over the skin presenting as grape-like nodules or singular arising from a nerve bundle in a deeper plane. An excision biopsy of one of these nodules should be adequate. The rest of them can be monitored unless symptomatic in any fashion.

Fibroma and histiocytoma are other types of benign masses that appear as rounded firm nodules of varying sizes in subcutaneous tissue. Complete local excision would be adequate. Malignant sarcomas can appear in the soft tissue to include liposarcoma, malignant histiocytoma, rhabdomyosarcoma, dermatofibrosarcoma, and angiosarcoma. These are rare abnormalities and require radical surgery and adjuvant therapy.

Synovial cysts can arise from the tendon sheaths, presenting as ganglions at the wrist or as a Baker's cyst in the popliteal area. These are noted at the specific locations and have a soft, fluctuant feel.

Bone tumors such as osteomas can look like sebaceous cysts or dermoids in appearance, but they are fixed to the bone and totally nonmobile on palpation.

Enlarged lymph nodes can present as subcutaneous masses. They can be infection-related, primary lymphomas, or metastatic disease. A careful search is made to detect the primary cause and by doing fine-needle aspiration (FNA) or biopsies.

Metastatic malignancy can appear as subcutaneous nodules. The primary can be in the breast, lung, or internal organs. A biopsy of one of the lesions will confirm the pathology.

KEY POINTS

Subcutaneous lumps are usually benign and can be excised with caution in the outpatient setting.

CHAPTER 62

Ganglion Cyst

INTRODUCTION

Ganglion cysts are connected to synovial sheaths when the fluid leaks out and solidifies as a partially encapsulated jelly-like material but is still connected to the tendon sheath or joint space. Most of them are seen around the wrist, even though they can occur around the finger, knee, or ankle. They are benign and can be left alone; however, many patients seek excision due to discomfort and cosmetic concerns.

DIAGNOSIS AND TREATMENT

Ganglion cysts are benign synovial cysts usually presenting around the wrist as a soft, mildly fluctuant, rounded, and well-defined mass. They can also occur around the ankle. Synovial cysts occurring at other areas are called bursa. It is a Baker's cyst when appearing behind the knee.

The ganglion cysts have a jelly-like material inside and cannot be aspirated for cure. They are connected to the carpal joints or to the tendon sheaths. They are painless but may cause a certain amount of tiredness when using the joint frequently. Small cysts can be observed without interventions, since they are benign and some of them can disappear spontaneously. Surgery is done if they are symptomatic or if the patient requests for cosmetic concerns.

Surgical excision is the best treatment. At surgery, a complete excision of the cyst is attempted, but they will commonly rupture toward the area where the tendon sheath is exposed. A glistening tendon is noted at the base. It is best to leave this area open to reduce recurrence. The skin and subcutaneous tissues are closed, and a mildly compressive bandage is applied.

KEY POINTS

Ganglion cysts are benign synovial cysts usually occurring in the wrist area. A complete excision is the best treatment.

CHAPTER 63

Skin and Subcutaneous Infections

■ INTRODUCTION

Patients frequently present to the emergency room or offices with urgent request to treat painful infected areas throughout the body. Many of them can be urgently treated with simple office procedures. However, many others will need admission to hospital and require wide radical surgery. Some of these can turn out to be life-threatening infections. Wound care is a subject by itself and becomes an integral part of their treatment.

■ CELLULITIS

Cellulitis represents the initial stage of subcutaneous infection, presenting as a reddened, warm, thickened, and painful area on the skin next to a site of insult. There is no pus formation yet. There is no fluctuation or abscess noticeable. The borders merge with the normal skin in a gradual fashion. At this phase, it is best to withhold any surgery or drainage procedures unless the site of injury or insult warrants an intervention, such as a foreign body implanted at the site. Antibiotics are given, along with tetanus toxoid, if there is documented injury as the cause. Moist compression is applied. It is best to avoid applying any topical agents. The area is marked and monitored daily for evidence of expansion or regression.

■ LYMPHANGITIS

Lymphangitis is a manifestation of infection spreading through lymphatic channels. Long streaks of reddish lines are seen under the skin extending from the site of infection to the regional lymph node, more visible under fair skin. Antibiotic therapy is needed to control the infection, most of which are staph or strep bacteria. It may go on to develop into regional abscesses.

■ ABSCESS

During this phase, the infection has become localized, with collection of pus and necrotic tissue inside the abscess cavity. It presents as a painful swelling with well-defined outer boundaries. Very often, it is an infected sebaceous cyst, where a preexisting sebaceous cyst gets infected. Sometimes, the abscess can break open and start leaking purulent material through the area. The initiating cause could be an insect bite or injury. Other causes are pilonidal cysts, perianal abscess, cat scratch disease, or diabetic infections. Internal abscesses such as subdiaphragmatic, hepatic, appendiceal, diverticular, and splenic abscesses are possible due to corresponding infections that get localized. Once the abscess has formed, it must be drained. On the skin and subcutaneous tissue, they are best incised widely and drained under sterile precautions. Any foreign body is removed, and the wound is debrided. If there is a cyst wall, it is removed. Usually, the cavity is packed with iodoform gauze strip loosely, and the wound is left open. Appropriate antibiotic therapy is initiated, and daily wound care is provided.

■ CARBUNCLE

In this situation, the infected area has multiple tiny abscesses spreading under the skin and subcutaneous tissue instead of a well-localized single abscess. The area looks inflamed, red, and tender. Multiple small pinhole-like areas exude a small amount of pus or inflammatory fluids. Many patients are diabetic; others may give a history of insect bites or minor trauma. Cultures may show multiple bacteria, but mostly they are staph or strep infections. The possibility of methicillin-resistant *Staphylococcus aureus* (MRSA) is high. These patients need open wide incision and debridement of all infected tissue to a healthy bleeding and uninfected level. The wound is usually packed with iodoform packing and left open for secondary closure.

NECROTIZING SOFT-TISSUE INFECTION

This could very well be the most dangerous subcutaneous or soft-tissue infection. Often, it starts as a small focus of infection but rapidly spreads through the soft-tissue planes and muscle planes, causing much larger destruction than what is visible from the exterior. There is often a mixed flora of both aerobic and anaerobic bacteria involved.

A variant of such an infection is often referred to as "flesh eating bacterial infection," which is caused by *Vibrio vulnificus*, a marine-based organism. The infection results from a seemingly minor skin puncture at the beach or lake, which rapidly becomes a lethal infection spreading through the extremity, along with fever and septic shock.

High suspicion and early aggressive treatment are required. Wide radical debridement with opening of tissue planes along with broad-spectrum antibiotic therapy is recommended. Systemic cardiorespiratory support and close monitoring are needed. Patients may need repeated surgical debridement to healthy bleeding tissue, excising all devitalized tissue.

GAS GANGRENE

As the term gas gangrene denotes, it is caused by a gas-forming organism, *Clostridium perfringens*, which is anaerobic gram-positive cocci. Most commonly, it occurs after trauma to the extremity. There is a rapid spread of the infection through muscle planes, and due to the anaerobic nature, there is destruction of muscle tissues. There is marked swelling, bleb formation, and onset of wet gangrene. The patient looks toxic with fever and shock. A plain X-ray of the area will show gas bubbles in tissue planes.

This would be considered a surgical emergency. Patients are taken for immediate open surgery when an amputation of the extremity is often needed due to the extent of tissue damage. The cut infected muscles will look purple and flabby with no blood flow and no contractions. The amputation may have to be extended to a higher level until healthy bleeding muscle tissue is noted.

DIABETIC INFECTIONS

Patients with diabetes mellitus are prone to developing deep soft-tissue infections. They have associated peripheral vascular disease and neuropathy. Often, the initial cause is a seemingly minor injury, such as careless nail pairing, insect bite, trauma to, foot from stepping on sharp objects, or scrapes and lacerations. Very often, the visible area of infection is deceptively small, while a larger necrotic area can be brewing underneath. Due to loss of sensation and ischemia, the patient may not be feeling much pain or other symptoms until it has progressed to a worse state. Diabetic involvement of joint in the ankle or foot can lead to deformities related to Charcot's disease, adding to the aggravation of the infected area. A high degree of suspicion is needed to undertake early intervention. This includes wide incision and debridement of the infected tissues, systemic antibiotics of broad-spectrum nature, and correction of ischemia of the limb.

DECUBITUS ULCERS

Decubitus ulcers are pressure sores noted over pressure points in nonambulatory and bedridden patients. Such pressure points include heels, presacral, and trochanteric areas. Due to constant pressure over these areas, the skin breaks down due to ischemia and subsequently, deeper tissue necrosis develops and secondary infection sets in. Some of the ulcers can become very large and deep, extending to joints and bones. Patients may not complain of symptoms but can develop fever and sepsis. It is important to provide preventive decubitus care to all nonambulatory patients. This includes frequent turning of the body, heel pads, waterbeds, and careful daily inspections. Once deep necrosis has developed, the wounds need to be debrided and antibiotics are given based on culture and sensitivity. Wound care may need to be continued for several weeks.

WOUND CARE

Long-term care of chronic wounds and nonhealing wounds is a topic by itself and has become a sub-specialty of general surgery. Many wound centers have been opened attached to hospitals.

The basic principles of management are similar in all these instances. The first step is to identify the underlying cause of the wound and the reason for the chronic nature of the wound. The next step is proper debridement of the wound to clean the base. At the same time, deep cultures are taken for appropriate antibiotic therapy. Then proper wound care is instituted, and follow-up care provided.

Acute infections, abscesses left open, infected wounds left open, and new-onset lacerations and abrasions have good prognosis compared to chronic nonhealing wounds. Some of the chronic wounds such as those secondary to lymphedema, obesity, and decubitus nature may not heal, and the goal is to keep them from getting worse.

All devitalized and necrotic tissue must be debrided to clean healthy base. Such debridement can be done using a conventional surgical scalpel, ultrasound devices, or hydrosurgery where high-pressure saline jets are used. Ultrasound and hydrojet are combined in Versajet. Such debridement often requires general or regional anesthesia.

Deep tissue cultures are taken to tailor appropriate antibiotic therapy. Topical antibiotics used are bacitracin, Neosporin, polymyxin, or neomycin. They may also need systemic antibiotic therapy.

The best solution to wash the wound is ordinary saline or water. It is best to avoid iodine-containing solutions or antiseptics at this phase.

The next step is placing moisturizing agents such as hydrogel or simply wet saline soaks. Many different commercial products and antibiotic ointments are promoted. Silver-containing hydrogel is Silvarov. Acquacel® Ag is calcium alginate.

Cell tissue products such as Epifix (MiMedx) can be obtained as powder, patches, or paste. Another powder is Prisma Promogran. Zinc oxide is helpful over erythematous borders. Silvadene is useful over burn sites.

An occlusive dressing is then applied. Sterile precautions, nontouch techniques, masks, and gloves are used, and often, an assistant is required to help.

Different types of dressing materials are available such as DuoDERM, Mepilex, or Hydrofera Blue with a foam containing gentian violet and methylene blue.

A major development in the field has been the use of wound vacuum-assisted closure (VAC). Wounds covered with wound VAC do not require daily dressings. The wound VAC is changed once every week. Commercially available products explain the step-wise application of the wound VAC. It is a very effective way of treating large open wounds. The vacuum drainage does allow a faster shrinkage of the wound. Disposable wound VAC, such as Praveena or tangential regional axial compression (TRAC) system, are options.

Direct coverage of skin loss can be done with Apligraf which is cultured skin from the prepuce of newborn or cadaveric skin or genetically prepared skin using stem cell technology. Autologous skin grafting is always an option.

KEY POINTS

Many skin and soft-tissue infections cause a great deal of alarm to the patient as being visible outside the body. Some of them can be minor and treated as office surgery, while some others can be more serious than what appears on the skin.

SECTION 10

Trauma

64. Lacerations
65. Stab Wounds
66. Gunshot Wounds
67. Blunt Injuries
68. Blast Injuries
69. Burns
70. Massive External Bleeding
71. Massive Internal Bleeding
72. Bites, Stings and Scrapes

CHAPTER 64

Lacerations

INTRODUCTION

All physicians should be able to provide first-aid care for the management of lacerations. They usually occur as a result of accidents or violence. It could be a clean-cut wound such as a knife injury or a very contaminated ragged wound such as a road accident. It can be a superficial abrasion with loss of skin as a patch or it can be deep, thus affecting the internal organs. Patients could come within a short time of the injury or a few days later after their own self-treatment has failed. All wounds must be evaluated, cleansed, and debrided. They should be closed primarily if it is safe.

EVALUATION AND MANAGEMENT

Emergency rooms and doctors' offices see patients with cuts, bruises, and skin lacerations. Patients expect any doctor to be able to help them with these urgent situations.

The first thing is to show empathy, calm the patient and family, and take them in for immediate care instead of making them wait. Even though the patient and family may be concerned about a laceration that is visible, the real serious problems could be internal, especially following automobile accidents. Hence, a complete history and physical examination must be done in all cases, irrespective of how small the external wound looks.

Evaluate the nature of the wound, causation, depth of the wound, size, bleeding, contamination, associated injuries, and options to close the wound. If there is massive bleeding, apply firm compression and a firm bandage, and call for surgical help to transfer the patient to an operating room. It is not easy to clamp the bleeding spot through the wound properly unless the bleeder is right in front of your eye.

Wash and cleanse the wound with running water or saline, and remove obvious foreign bodies and contaminations. Inject local anesthesia, give pain medication to the patient, and then work on the wound. Excise and debride devitalized tissues and repair the tissues loosely. If it is a clean-cut wound that happened <4 hours ago, it can be closed primarily. Contaminated wounds or that occurred >6 hours ago are better off left open or partially closed. Apply occlusive dressing.

Superficial abrasions and lacerations with small amount of skin loss can be left open as they will heal spontaneously over several days. An exception to this would be injuries to face and neck, where effort is made to achieve primary closure as best as possible because of cosmetic concerns. Blood supply is excellent to these areas to allow good healing.

If there are complex injuries underneath, make appropriate referrals. If there is gross contamination, do not close the skin; consider secondary closure at a later date. Use of antibiotics is considered for prophylaxis as well as for contamination.

KEY POINTS

Many superficial lacerations and wounds can be closed in the outpatient setting.

CHAPTER 65

Stab Wounds

INTRODUCTION

Injury following stab wounds or penetrating wounds by sharp instruments is more predictable compared to other types of injuries. The wound is visible on the outside, and the history will give information as to the type of instrument used and the direction or depth of infliction. The injury itself may be skin deep or into muscle, but internal organs could be damaged. Depending on the location, it can affect the pleura, lung, pericardium, intra-abdominal viscera, neck, deeper arteries, veins, or nerves.

EVALUATION AND MANAGEMENT

Penetrating wounds caused by sharp instruments such as a knife, machete, ice pick, sword, pencil, screwdriver, and such materials create problems anywhere from minor injuries to life-threatening serious wounds.

Often, there is a history of violence, where one person inflicts a wound on another. The injury site is visible and somewhat predictable in its course and seriousness.

Soft-tissue injuries to the extremities are less consequential compared to stab wounds of the abdomen or chest. Wounds directly overlying arteries or veins can cause serious hemorrhage. If there is massive arterial bleeding spurting from a stab wound site, the best course of action is to apply direct compression of the bleeding spot immediately and transfer the patient from the emergency room to the operating room. Under quick anesthesia, with minimal preparation and the wound extended while maintaining the direct compression, expose the artery proximally and apply proper vascular clamp and then do necessary repair under direct vision. This is far superior to blindly applying clamps and suturing in the emergency room.

Some of the stab wounds of the extremities can cause only venous injury, resulting in a large hematoma. If the arterial circulation is intact, many of them can be observed and may self-seal by tamponade. After a few days, the hematoma can be evacuated and wound packed, if necessary.

Some of the stab wounds can result in an arteriovenous fistula. A bruit can be heard at the site of injury. This will require surgical correction after full evaluation and investigation that includes a preoperative angiogram. Open surgical control of the artery above and below the injury is obtained first, and then the injury site is exposed carefully. The injured segment of artery and vein are repaired by appropriate techniques.

Stab wounds of the abdomen can be evaluated for internal damage and probably observed if superficial. A focused assessment with sonography in trauma (FAST) examination in the emergency room is acceptable, but it is better to avoid getting a computed tomography (CT) scan initially, which can delay emergency care of the patient. A wound examination and minimal exploration are acceptable if it looks superficial. If it looks deep, the best course of action would be a laparoscopic examination to assess the damage and perform necessary repair instead of doing routine laparotomy in all cases. Details of the repair at surgery will depend upon the findings. In general, bowel injuries following stab wounds can be primarily repaired.

Stab wounds over the chest need a chest X-ray. Most of them will initially need a chest tube placement. Massive bleeding or lung collapse will require thoracotomy. An injury over the precordium can be a pinhole if made with an ice pick or a screwdriver, but the damage could be serious to the heart and pericardium. Stab wounds over the precordium need to be evaluated for pericardial tamponade and cardiac injuries. An emergency thoracotomy may be needed.

Stab wounds of the neck should be formally explored for injuries of major arteries, veins, pharynx, larynx, and esophagus.

KEY POINTS

All stab wounds need careful evaluation for internal injuries. They may be simple or complicated.

CHAPTER 66

Gunshot Wounds

INTRODUCTION

Gunshot wounds can cause serious damage to internal organs and death. Gunshot wounds of the head, neck, and precordium are almost lethal. Abdominal gunshot wounds can often be saved. The velocity and size of the bullet are factors in the extent of damage. All gunshot wounds are treated with extreme urgency, irrespective of how the patient initially appears. A complete physical examination and X-rays are initially taken while starting resuscitative measures at the same time.

EVALUATION AND MANAGEMENT

Gunshot wounds kill an average of 50 people a day in the United States. These high-velocity missile injuries cause internal damages of a lethal nature in a very short time. They are caused by acts of violence, homicides, suicides, and accidents. An easy availability of a variety of weapons, stressful lifestyle, and culture issues lead to quick use of guns, even for trivial causes. Efforts to introduce gun control in the United States have so far failed.

When a patient with a gunshot is brought to the emergency room, immediate attention is given for quick stabilization, resuscitation, and assessment of all injuries.

Teamwork evaluation and treatment are done in a coordinated fashion. How many shots were fired into the body? Where are they located? What are their trajectories? Where are the entrance wounds? Where are the exit wounds? What are the vital signs? Is the person dead or alive? What are the possible internal damages? All these questions must be answered as quickly as possible.

If the gunshot wound is to the brain and the patient is already dead, there is often no point in going through extensive testing and supportive measures.

Gunshots into the chest cavity and abdominal cavity, on the other hand, must be resuscitated aggressively since most of them can be saved. Large-bore intravenous lines are inserted, preferably in separate extremities. The airway is protected, and the patient is intubated rapidly. A Foley catheter and nasogastric tubes are inserted in preparation for surgery. Blood is drawn for all laboratory works, including type and match for transfusions, drug profile, and coagulation screening.

Chest tubes are placed into the involved side of the chest cavity. There is no need to wait for a chest X-ray to verify hemothorax or pneumothorax. The chest X-rays can be obtained afterward. Do not send the patient for computed tomography (CT) scans initially, which will delay patient care in the critical moments.

Similarly, if the gunshot wound is into the pelvis or abdomen, it is best to take the patient to the operating room immediately for open exploratory laparotomy.

Extremity wounds should be evaluated for arterial, venous, and neurological deficits. Fractures and dislocations should be identified and splinted.

It is not important to remove the bullet, unlike a common myth, as shown in the movies. It is important to repair the injuries and correct damages.

The bullet wounds usually create an entrance wound and an exit wound. If an exit wound cannot be found and accounted for, then the bullet may be lodged inside the body and should be identified.

Exact repair depends upon the exact injury. The first priority is to stop the bleeding, wherever it may be. Injuries to the heart, major veins, and arteries need rapid exposure of the area and careful repair. Bowel, bladder, liver, and bile duct injuries need debridement of the edges and repair. Often, they can be repaired primarily. Sometimes, they may require diversions or secondary repairs. Bowel injuries usually have an even number of holes, accounting for entrance and exit. Look carefully at mesenteric side edges for injuries in the bowel if an exit wound cannot be found.

KEY POINTS

Gunshot wounds can be lethal and need immediate assessment and intervention.

CHAPTER 67

Blunt Injuries

INTRODUCTION

Blunt injuries are unpredictable to the extent of their damage. One must suspect internal injuries in all cases. Cerebral concussion, subdural hematoma, whiplash injury to the cervical spine, spinal cord injuries, fracture of the vertebrae, contusion of the lung, injury to the pancreas, mesenteric blood vessels, pelvic fractures, fracture of the long bones, and musculoskeletal injuries are all possibilities following falls or automobile accidents.

EVALUATION AND MANAGEMENT

Blunt injuries can be from a fall, an automobile accident, or a violent act with a blunt object such as a club or stick. These injuries can be minor, involving skin and muscle only, or they can be having serious internal injuries. As such, these patients need careful examination and evaluation. All patients are started on emergency precautions with attention to airway, breathing, cardiac care, intravenous fluid, laboratory work, and appropriate investigations, irrespective of how they appear on arrival.

Blunt injury to the head can result in a brain concussion, subdural or intracerebral hemorrhage, or a whiplash injury to the cervical spine. Examination of the neurological system and pupils and external signs such as bleeding from the ear or nose is assessed. A computed tomography (CT) scan of the brain is requested. A neurosurgeon is consulted as some of these patients will need emergency craniotomy.

Blunt injury to the chest can cause lung injury, fracture of the ribs, flail chest, pneumothorax, or injury to the pulmonary vessels. An X-ray of the chest and a CT scan of the chest are requested. Sudden deceleration can cause aortic root or arch dissection, which will be seen as widening of mediastinum on a regular chest X-ray. CT angiogram is done for confirmation, and a cardiothoracic surgeon is consulted.

Blunt injury to the abdomen can lead to a variety of internal damages. Injury to the liver and spleen or mesenteric vessels can cause intra-abdominal hemorrhage. A focused assessment with sonography for trauma (FAST) evaluation is done in the emergency room.

One of the rapid deceleration injuries to the abdomen is related to seat belt compressing across the mid abdomen. Injury to the pancreas or transection of the body of the pancreas can occur. A CT scan of the abdomen and pelvis is done. Initial laparoscopic assessment followed by open surgery will be needed to control the bleeding or repair the damage.

A fracture of the pelvis can result in large pelvic bleeding that may require interventional radiology assistance to selectively embolize the bleeding arteries. Retroperitoneal injury to the kidneys or great vessels can happen. A CT scan of the abdomen will be required in these cases for better evaluation. All midline retroperitoneal hematomas must be explored to rule out major vessel injuries. Lateral hematomas and pelvic hematomas can be observed since exploration may cause more damage than allowing tamponade effect by nature.

Falls from height can result in vertebral fractures, coccygeal fractures, impalement injuries, and long bone fractures. Spinal cord injuries resulting in paraplegia or quadriplegia can occur. X-rays of spine and magnetic resonance imaging (MRI) are done, and emergency treatment measures as per neurosurgery opinion are instituted. In case of cervical spine injuries, care is taken to avoid movement of the neck by using neck braces.

KEY POINTS

Blunt injuries can be lethal or minor. They need careful evaluation, workup, observation, and cannot be taken lightly even if there are no visible injury marks outside.

CHAPTER 68

Blast Injuries

INTRODUCTION

International terrorism and modern-day warfare have brought potential for blast injuries everywhere. They bring a combination of loud noise, burns, and high-velocity flying objects, resulting in large, contaminated wounds and unpredictable internal and external injuries. Improvised explosive devices (IEDs) have glass pieces, nails, screws, and gunpowder mixed in. Sharp objects can lodge inside the body with almost invisible external wounds.

EVALUATION AND MANAGEMENT

With the changing times, newer modes of attacks and terrorism have become common across the globe. The perpetrators want to create fear and anxiety.

Sometimes, bombs are exploded in crowded places; sometimes, these IEDs are left in a car or a bag. Bombs explode as part of military warfare, causing injuries to many civilians as well as soldiers. Sometimes, they are suicide bombers. The explosion can be in open space or inside of the buildings. They can also occur as a result of accidents in factories or festivals using fireworks. IEDs contain many sharp particles such as nails, screws, glass pieces, and other sharp projectiles mixed with gunpowder or other explosives. This results in numerous sharp flying objects that cause varying penetrating injuries to people standing nearby.

Blast injuries are a combination of penetrating injuries, blunt injuries, burns, crush injuries, and mangling of whole-body parts.

The injuries caused can vary from a superficial laceration to a very deep internal wound that may not get recognized for a long time. The external injury may look like nothing more than a pinhole, but a flying nail, sharp object, or shrapnel can be lodged in the aorta or lung. Sometimes, there can be multiple sharp and blunt objects buried in different parts of the body such as glass pieces, screws, bolts, gunpowder, and chemicals.

One of the injuries noted from the heavy blast is perforation of ear drum and resulting hearing loss. Blast lung injury can present as lung contusion and hypoxia. Intestinal contusions, submucosal hemorrhage, and delayed perforations can occur. Extremities can be mangled or crushed, with fractures and large open wounds with charred and burnt tissues.

The important thing is to remember that blast injuries can be very unpredictable and cannot be taken lightly. Every patient must be thoroughly examined, X-rayed, and investigated with a computed tomography (CT) scan for internal injuries. There may be associated burn injuries of the skin or chemical injuries.

Treatment consists of cleansing and removing obvious protruding foreign bodies, IV fluids, antibiotics, and corrective measures to handle internal injuries. Surgery may involve amputation of mangled extremities, laparotomy for intra-abdominal injuries, thoracotomy for thoracic wounds, or even craniotomy for head injuries. Many patients will need intensive care monitoring and multisystem support.

Blast injuries create logistic problems of mass disasters since many patients will be injured at the same time. Triage of the sickest and urgent operations will have to be prioritized. Staffing, resources, operating facilities, and transportation to the surrounding hospitals are challenges to be met.

KEY POINTS

Blast injuries can be tricky and need immediate attention to full details. Careful evaluation for internal injuries is needed.

CHAPTER 69

Burns

INTRODUCTION

Two important factors to consider in treating burns are the depth of the burn and body surface area involved. The depth of the burn is characterized as first-, second-, and third-degree burns. Body surface area is measured by the rule of nines. Over 30% of body surface burn carries a high mortality, and they should be sent to special burn centers if possible. Rapid fluid management is critical in the immediate care of burns to save lives.

EVALUATION AND MANAGEMENT

Burns are one reason for patients to be brought to the emergency room. The history is evidently given as to what happened, the time of the incident, how it happened, and what was involved. The most common cause is flames and scalds from cooking accidents.

Two main concerns from the medical point of view are the depth of the burn and the surface area involved.

Depth of the burn is described as first degree, which means superficial epidermis only; second degree, which means full thickness of the skin; or third degree, which means full thickness of the skin and subcutaneous tissue is involved. A fourth-degree burn involves deeper tissues such as bones, muscles, and internal organs. The depth of the burn can be assessed by the appearance of the wound, touch sensation, pain felt by the patient, appearance of hair follicles, and bleb formation.

A first-degree burn is painful for the patient, painful to touch, erythematous, and blanches to touch. It involves only the outer layer of the epidermis.

A second-degree burn has a combination of injury to the epidermis and dermis; some areas of second-degree burns may have superficial blisters but still retain touch and pain sensations. Some areas may have extension to the reticular layer with pallor, but it is still painful, and hair follicles are retained. Upon opening the blisters, pink base is visible.

A third-degree burn extends through both the epidermis and dermis to the subcutaneous tissue. It looks like charred, grayish, and open leathery tissue with no bleeding, no hair, and no sensation.

The treatment depends upon the degree of burns. First- and second-degree burns can heal spontaneously with time and local care. However, third-degree burns require debridement and excision of the dead tissues with skin grafting. If they are causing compartment syndrome, arterial or venous compromise due to circumferential burn of the extremity, then immediate escharotomy is done by incising on the eschar, longitudinally deep to bleeding level tissue.

The size of the burn is also a critical factor. The rule of nines is often used to measure the surface area of the burn involved. In adults, the face is 9%, each front and back of each upper extremity is 9%, each front and back of each lower extremity is 18%, front of torso is 18%, back of torso is 18%, and perineum and genitalia will take up 1% to make it a total of 100% **(Fig. 69.1)**.

Burns involving >30% of the body surface must be immediately transferred to a special burn center after starting intravenous (IV) fluids per protocol and after providing first-aid care. Other patients can be handled in a regular hospital.

Emergency resuscitation involves starting an IV fluid rapidly to overcome dehydration, shock, and renal shutdown. The Parkland formula is usually used to calculate initial fluid requirement. It is 4 mL of lactated Ringer's solution per kilogram body weight per percent total body surface area burned. Half of this amount is administered within the first

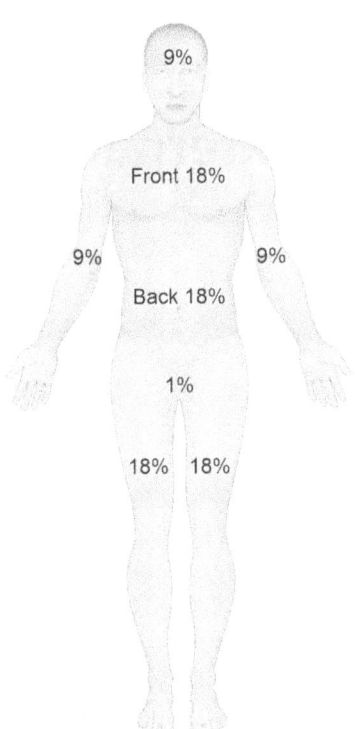

Fig. 69.1: Rule of nines to estimate body surface of burn.

BOX 69.1: Burn care.

- *Fluid replacement*—Parkland formula—4 mL/kg wt per % of burn area. Half of it is given in first 8 hours and the rest within 24 hours. Many other formulae are available
- *Calorie requirement*—1,500 K calories per % of burn area per 24 hours
- *Monitoring*—vital signs, urine output, renal function tests, pulmonary state, all other organ functions. Look out for inhalation injury
- *Wound care applications*—silver sulfadiazine (silvadene), bacitracin, neomycin, polymyxin, silver nitrate soaks, 0.025% sodium hypochlorite (Dakin's solution), 0.25% acetic acid
- *Wound coverings*—Vaseline gauze, Opsite, Biobrane, TransCyte, Integra, Pig skin graft, Allograft from cadaveric skin, split-thickness autograft
- *Wound surgery*—debridement, escharotomy, tangential excision, full-thickness excision, prevention or correction of contractures

---

8 hours and the rest within 24 hours. Careful monitoring of vital signs and urine output is set up.

Local care of the wound with Vaseline® gauze and topical application of Silvadene® (silver sulfadiazine) is done. Other options are bacitracin, neomycin, or silver nitrate soaks. Opsite coverings can help as dressings. Antibiotics are withheld until infection is noted. Pain medication is best given as IV morphine **(Box 69.1)**.

Further therapy may be needed to avoid contractures and wound coverage with skin grafting and rehabilitation. Inhalation injury should be watched for in all burn cases.

Inhalation of smoke, heat, and toxic fumes can cause significant tracheobronchial-pulmonary injury, requiring use of ventilatory support, nebulizers, and antibiotics. Smoke inhalation injury can lead to death, even when the surface burn is negligent.

A completely different topic is burns caused by chemicals. It can be caustic materials such as acid, alkali, or poisonous material spilled or thrown on the body or such chemicals ingested out of ignorance or suicide attempts. Extrinsic burns caused by chemicals are treated with the same principles as heat burns. Washing the area profusely with water is the first step. Ingested chemicals cause stricture of esophagus, esophagitis, gastritis, or perforations.

Yet, another category is electrical burns and lightning accidents. Patients can sustain remote injuries related to grounding the electric current or cardiac arrest and death.

KEY POINTS

The depth of the burn and surface area of the burn are two critical evaluations to be made. Immediate IV fluid replacement per protocol is needed in all major burns.

Chapter 70: Massive External Bleeding

INTRODUCTION

Visible blood loss is scary, and even simple first-aid measures can be lifesaving. Similar to initiating cardiopulmonary resuscitation (CPR) in cardiac arrest or the Heimlich maneuver in choking, "stop the bleeding" is another phrase used in emergency care in the field of injury. This includes applying direct pressure over the bleeding spot, applying tight bandages, applying tourniquets above the bleeding spot, and transporting patients to the nearest healthcare facility.

EVALUATION AND MANAGEMENT

"Stop the bleeding" is a newly adopted first-aid phrase by the American College of Surgeons to teach patients, doctors, and the general public in controlling massive external bleeding in an effort to save lives. In many situations, where there are gunshot wounds, acts of violence, or accidents, massive bleeding can be noted and stopped by timely intervention. This can save many lives.

Actions at the scene can be critical. These involve applying direct pressure over the bleeding area with fingers, gauze pads, and towels, applying a tourniquet just above the bleeding spot, calling for ambulance or police for emergency help, requesting others in helping to initiate CPR if necessary, and transporting patients to the medical facility.

Once the patient has reached the emergency room, the same above-mentioned initial measures are established. In addition, one would start the best intravenous (IV) fluids, send blood for type and cross-match, and call for immediate transport of the patient to the operating room under the guidance of a qualified surgeon.

Once the patient is in the operating room, immediate awake intubation is done, protecting against aspiration. Rapid preparation and draping of the extremity or body segment are done while maintaining compression to the bleeding spot. An incision is made above and below this site to rapidly expose the main artery above and below the wound. The surgeon must know the anatomy and exposure techniques of various arterial and venous pathways. Once the proximal artery is identified, a proper vascular clamp is applied. Then compression is released, and careful dissection of the depth of the wound is made.

The exact nature of the injury must be identified, and then appropriate repair of the bleeding site is accomplished. These wounds are usually contaminated. All devitalized tissues are debrided. Ragged and unhealthy edges are trimmed. If the artery can be primarily closed, such as in clean knife injury, then it can be done. Otherwise, an interposition graft will be needed. One should not anastomose an artery under tension. This will break down soon with another episode of massive bleeding. The ideal graft is a reversed autogenous saphenous vein since synthetic grafts can get infected.

Another option to consider is placement of temporary shunts between proximal and distal cut ends of the artery to reestablish the circulation. Anticoagulants are given to prevent clot formation. Any orthopedic injuries that require bone stabilization can be done at this time before the final arterial graft placement. If needed, patients can be transported from field hospitals to tertiary care hospitals with the shunt in place. This is one of the strategies used in war wounds, where patients are stabilized in the field hospital and then transported over to the base hospital.

Massive external bleeding can happen due to complications from surgical procedures and endovascular interventions. With the advent of laparoscopic and robotic procedures, chances of injuring arterial structures have also increased, from the port placements to dissections close to arteries. Following cardiac catheterizations, endovascular valve replacements and aneurysm repairs, chance of bleeding from large access sites, resulting in expanding hematoma and false aneurysm formation, can happen.

Another situation where massive bleeding can take place is in the operating room itself while performing another surgery. It can happen during any surgery, but laparoscopic procedures have brought another set of problems too. Classic situations are when there is cystic artery bleeding during laparoscopic cholecystectomy, splenic artery bleeding during splenectomy, iliac artery bleeding during pelvic surgery, aortic injury or vena cava injury during port placement, femoral artery or popliteal artery bleedings during hip or knee surgery, excessive bleeding during vascular surgery procedures, and so forth.

In all these occasions, immediate control of the bleeding is critical. If the bleeding area can be clearly seen and can be clipped safely, then one may make one attempt to do so. Otherwise, the best option is to open the abdomen immediately instead of wasting time and clipping organs poorly visible in a pool of blood. Once the abdomen is open, apply direct pressure with lap pads, expose the area with retractors, precisely identify the exact bleeding spot, and then place vascular sutures or ligatures to stop the bleeding. Arrangements should be made for adequate fluid replacement and blood transfusion at the same time.

KEY POINTS

Initial immediate actions at the scene of the accident can save lives. Apply pressure or a tourniquet to stop the bleeding and transport the patient to an operating room as quickly as possible. Immediate exposure of the main artery above the bleeding spot with proper application of a vascular clamp with subsequent careful repair is the best treatment.

Massive Internal Bleeding

INTRODUCTION

Massive internal bleeding can happen following any type of trauma such as stab wounds, gunshot wounds, automobile accidents, or falls. It can also be a spontaneous internal hemorrhage following ruptured abdominal aortic aneurysms (AAA) or any other visceral aneurysms, ruptured ectopic pregnancy, ruptured liver tumors, or spontaneous or delayed rupture of spleen. Another common reason is postoperative hemorrhage following any type of abdominal or pelvic surgery. This is more so with the advent of laparoscopic surgery. The patient can go into rapid hypotension and hypovolemic shock. It is lifesaving to make a quick diagnosis and immediate open surgery to stop the bleeding.

EVALUATION AND MANAGEMENT

Massive internal bleeding should be suspected when there is a history of trauma or if there is unexplained hypotension. This may be obvious in gunshot wounds or stab wounds. It may not be obvious following automobile accidents or falls. Sometimes, the fall or accident may have been a few days ago.

Causes of nontraumatic conditions that lead to internal hemorrhage are ruptured AAA, ruptured ectopic pregnancy, ruptured splenic artery aneurysm, or spontaneous rupture of the spleen or liver related to tumors or enlargements.

Another common cause of internal hemorrhage is postoperative bleeding following any type of abdominal surgery. This is more so after complex vascular surgery such as aortic or iliac artery procedures, liver or spleen resections, or pelvic surgery for cancers. Laparoscopic surgery and robotic surgery have brought another set of reasons for massive internal bleeding. It can be situations such as cystic artery bleeding after laparoscopic cholecystectomy, splenic artery bleeding following upper abdominal surgery, or uterine artery bleeding after hysterectomy. During the initial port placement, bleeding can happen from the aorta, vena cava, or mesenteric vessels but is not identified immediately due to vasospasm and mesenteric coverage of the area.

The patient usually presents in hypovolemic shock with associated abdominal distension or back pain. In cases of trauma, a history of such an incident is available. In certain cases, the history of trauma may have been a few days ago as in the case of delayed rupture of the spleen. Associated fracture of lower ribs on the left side with left shoulder pain should lead to suspicion of splenic tear.

A focused assessment with sonography in trauma (FAST) examination in the emergency room will show fluid in the abdominal cavity and a computed tomography (CT) scan or ultrasound can corroborate the findings.

Immediate resuscitation includes sending blood for type and match, starting large-bore intravenous (IV), and transferring the patient to an operating room as soon as possible.

At surgery, a long midline laparotomy incision is made, quick autotransfusion arrangements are made, blood is suctioned out, and the abdomen is packed with lap pads all around. An initial quick assessment is made as to which general area the bleeding is welling from. Go systematically to look in the pelvis, retroperitoneum (**Fig. 71.1**), right upper quadrant (RUQ), or left upper quadrant (LUQ).

Once the general area of bleeding is recognized, lap pad compression is once again placed in that section, proper exposure is obtained, and the rest of the bowels are retracted away after removing unwanted lap pads. Then a focused search for the actual cause of bleeding is made. Once the exact site of the bleeding is identified, that area is compressed selectively and arrangements are made to stop it. Sometimes, this may just be a finger pressure or a clamp application.

If the spleen is the cause of the bleeding, then the spleen should be mobilized from its bed and brought to the surface before attempting a total or partial splenectomy.

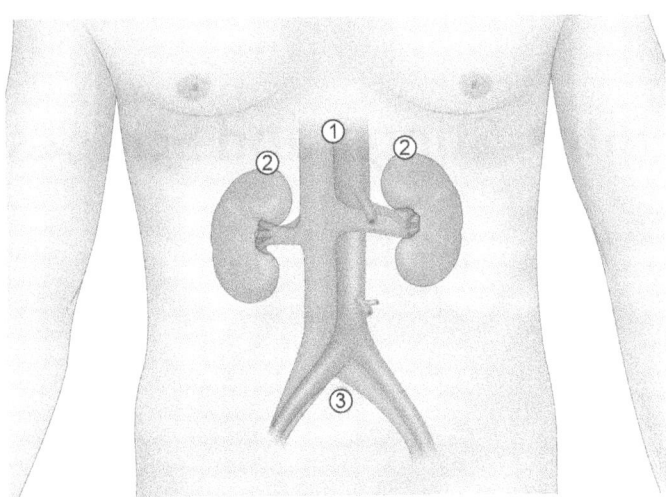

Fig. 71.1: Zones of retroperitoneal hematoma.
Zone 1: Hematoma must be explored to rule out injuries to great vessels in retroperitoneum aorta, vena cava, etc.
Zone 2: Flank hematoma in retroperitoneum, usually due to kidney injuries, can be explored or observed with caution.
Zone 3: Pelvic hematomas are best left unexplored to maintain the tamponade effect.

If it is a ruptured ectopic pregnancy, the involved ovary and fallopian tubes are pinched between fingers and a clamp is applied across the pedicle. They would require a unilateral salpingectomy with or without oophorectomy.

If it is a ruptured AAA, the retroperitoneum is opened along the midline, the neck of the aortic aneurysm is identified and mobilized, and an aortic clamp is applied. If it is not easy, then the aorta is immediately clamped at the diaphragmatic level. To do this, one should insert a nasogastric tube to feel the esophagus. Dissection is made to the right side of the esophagus at the crus of diaphragm, with the crural fibers sharply divided or separated to feel the aortic pulsation.

If it is the liver that is bleeding, the first step is to pack and apply compression. Then identify the exact area of the bleeding. Pringle maneuver is pinching the free border of the lesser omentum through the foramen of Winslow, where the hepatic artery, portal vein, and common bile duct (CBD) are located going toward the liver. If the bleeding is massive and persistent, then a limited liver resection is needed, exposing the bleeding site in the area of resection. At times, bleeding from the back side of liver from hepatic veins or from the depth of liver is difficult to control. Firm compression with firm packing may be the only temporary solution.

Bleeding from major veins in the abdomen can be lethal and much more problematic than arterial bleeding. This includes bleeding from vena cava, portal vein, hepatic veins, and superior mesenteric vein. Major veins cannot be clamped since they easily tear and bleed more. The first step is to apply compression directly over the area with a fingertip or a gauze pad. Using bulky nontraumatic forceps and finger pressure, the exact bleeding spot is identified. Sutures are quickly placed with fine Prolene sutures.

Intrathoracic bleeding needs an immediate thoracotomy. Control of lung hilum with suture of the bleeding vessel is done if it is arising from hilar vessels. It could be bleeding from heart, aorta, or major vessels.

It is important to have good help, teamwork, good exposure, and good instruments to get good results in controlling massive internal hemorrhage.

In certain situations, an interventional radiologist may be able to provide backup by selective embolization in the pelvis, mesenteric, and nonaccessible vessels above the mandible or at the thoracic outlet.

Patients with massive hemorrhage can easily go into hypothermia, acidosis, coagulation failure, and electrolyte imbalance. Correction of these with good anesthesia backup and transfusion are needed measures.

KEY POINTS

Massive internal hemorrhage carries high mortality or morbidity. Quick and efficient teamwork can save lives.

CHAPTER 72

Bites, Stings, and Scrapes

INTRODUCTION

Patients present to the emergency room, outpatient clinic, or offices of doctors with complaints of a variety of apparent minor injuries resulting from bites, stings, or scrapes caused by animals, insects, or even plants. Some of these may turn out to be life-threatening, even though the site of injury may look small. Snakebites and dog bites cause a great deal of fear and panic. It is important to evaluate them carefully with a methodical plan of treatment.

SNAKEBITES

Snakebites are a common injury in rural areas and in tropical countries, more often in farming or forested areas. Many misconceptions have been perpetuated for generations in providing initial care of these victims. Examples are application of tight tourniquets above the site of bite or incising and sucking the area of bite to let out the poison, or application of plant-based pastes over the site. None of these measures are of any value and may in fact cause more damage than good.

Effort is made to identify the snake to know if it is poisonous or not. Bystanders or neighboring local people may be of assistance. If one is certain that it is a nonpoisonous snake, then no further treatment is necessary other than observation of the bite area and the systemic status of the patient. Inspection of the bite mark may give some clues. Generally, two puncture wounds at the bite site are from poisonous snakes. Redness, swelling, and severe pain also indicate poisonous snakes. If one is certain that it is a poisonous snake, or if an identification cannot be made with certainty, then the patient is admitted for observation, started on maintenance intravenous fluid, the bite area is marked with a marker circularly, and frequent vital signs are recorded. Wash the area with soap and water and keep the limb immobile or above heart level. Antivenin injection is administered per protocol as soon as possible. Follow the recommended schedule by poison control agency.

There are two types of major reactions that the venom can cause—hemolytic reaction and neurotoxic reaction. If a patient goes into hemolytic reaction, then blood transfusion is arranged. If neurotoxicity is observed, then continued administration of antivenin to maximum dosage is given along with corticosteroids, anticonvulsants, and antihistamines. If the patient goes into multiple organ failure, then full-throttle multisystem support including ventilator assistance is set up.

Surgery on the bite area is considered if there is compartment syndrome or necrosis of the tissue. The bite area is marked and carefully observed for the next several hours and days. If there is evidence of tissue necrosis, immediate wide excision of the devitalized tissue is done to prevent further extension of necrosis and wound is left open with moist saline dressings.

SCORPION STINGS

Out of 1,500 different species of scorpions, only about 30 are poisonous. Hence, vast majority of scorpion stings do not need any treatment. Stings by scorpions can occur in rural areas and camping sites near forests. Scorpions are nocturnal animals and do not sting unless provoked or attacked. The venom is carried in its tail and can be dangerous for children and elders. The venom is neurotoxic and can also lead to allergic reactions.

Appearance of the sting site looks like a pin prick initially, which later can become very painful and red. The wound site is marked and carefully observed for increasing local symptoms. Patients are also observed for any systemic symptoms such as tachycardia, sweating, nausea, vomiting, muscle twitching, irritability, and dyspnea.

Local treatment includes application of ice and cold compress and immobilization of the body part. If secondary infections occur or if tissue necrosis is noted, antibiotics are administered, and local debridement of the necrotic tissue is done. Systemic treatment with antivenom is started immediately if systemic symptoms are noted, with particular emphasis on children and older adults. Sedation, antihistamines, and systemic support are considered as the situation demands.

SPIDER BITES

Out of many different species of spiders, only two are dangerous—black widow spider and brown recluse spider. These two carry venoms that can cause local tissue damage and systemic symptoms.

Initially, the bite area looks like a red, raised bump with itchy sensation. The pain increases over the next several hours, and the center becomes pale and then dark blue with a reddish ring around it. The area develops deep necrosis and breaks open with an ulceration and blister formation. The patients may also develop fever, chills, abdominal cramps, nausea, vomiting, tachycardia, and dyspnea.

Local care initially is to wash with soap and water and cool compressive soaks. Antihistamine and analgesics are prescribed. No antivenom treatment is used routinely. Systemic antibiotics and supportive care are rendered. The area will need wide incision drainage and debridement of all necrotic tissue. The wound is left open with wet saline soaks for secondary closure over several days.

DOG BITES

India has too many stray dogs on the streets, and dog bites and related complications are common occurrences. The greatest danger from bites of dogs and wild animals is transmission of rabies, which is a lethal viral infection. Most dogs are not infected with rabies, but it is difficult to be certain until the dog is observed for at least 2 weeks for symptoms of rabies, by which time the victim may become incurable.

Rabies is caused by *Lyssavirus*, which is stored in the salivary gland of the animal. Transmission occurs when the infected saliva is inoculated at the bite area or if the saliva is spilled onto mucous membranes or eyes of the victim even without an actual bite. Rabies causes a wide variety of cerebral and neurological symptoms such as agitation, hallucinations, anxiety, and paralysis. There is severe spasm of esophagus and larynx, leading to difficulty in swallowing (hydrophobia) and alteration of voice, which is interpreted as a bark by common man.

Initial local treatment of the wound is provided with washing the area with copious amounts of soap and water and with betadine solution. Debridement of devitalized tissue is done, and wounds are left open with moist saline dressings.

Systemic treatment with prophylactic rabies vaccine is started immediately, along with human rabies immunoglobulin. Usually, 7 days of therapy with vaccination is recommended for satisfactory prophylaxis. Once the actual symptoms of rabies occur, there will be very little hope for recovery.

HUMAN BITES

This may sound funny as a topic included along with various animal bites. However, human bites can also cause severe tissue damage. Human bites can occur as part of a fight or violence between individuals. A punch on the face can end up with an injury on the knuckles from the teeth. Human bites can be classified as occlusion bite injuries secondary to actual bite of the body or as closed fist injury, where the dorsal side of the metacarpophalangeal joint is injured in a fist fight. Human saliva contains mixed aerobic and anerobic bacteria, and *Eikenella corrodens*. If the injury is deep, the bacteria can spread through the tendon sheath.

Initial symptoms are intense pain and noticeable wound at the site of injury, followed by redness, pus formation, and fever and chills.

The wound is immediately cleansed with copious amounts of soap and water and betadine solution and occlusive dressing is applied. Systemic antibiotics are started immediately and continued for 1 week. Amoxicillin-clavulanate, cipro, and clindamycin are choices. The patient may need extensive debridement with assistance of the hand surgeon if tendon injury is suspected.

Possibility of transmission of herpes, hepatitis, and human immunodeficiency virus (HIV) infection is kept in mind.

MOSQUITO BITE

Mosquito bites are not directly affecting the surgeon's clinic or practice since the wound inflicted by the mosquito is very small. However, the surgeon is to be aware of the variety of surgical problems created by the illnesses caused by mosquitoes. Mosquito-borne infections include malaria, filariasis, yellow fever, dengue, chikungunya, zika, West Nile virus, and encephalitis.

Patients with malaria can present to the surgeon with enlarged spleen, filariasis can present as unilateral non-pitting edema of extremity, and dengue and chikungunya as arthritic pain. Treatment depends on the individual situation. Prevention of mosquito bite by using mosquito nets, screens, disinfectants, repellents, and other public health measures are useful measures.

STINGRAYS

Stingrays are marine animals that float in shallow water. They are flat, smooth and silky, dark, flat fan-like fish with a tail, often seen in tropical and subtropical areas. They can be hiding in the sand and move away from any disturbances or vibrations. People are advised to shuffle their feet in the shallow waters in coastal areas instead of stepping in it. Stingrays have sharp cartilaginous spines with venom. When a person accidentally steps on them, the spine can break off and make deep cuts with broken pieces of the spine embedded in the wound.

Patients complain of intense pain, with a sting mark on the skin, which can become red and inflamed. They could develop systemic symptoms of nausea, vomiting, diarrhea, muscle cramps, and secondary infections. Marine-oriented bacteria can cause severe necrotizing infections.

The area is cleansed with profuse amounts of hot water, as hot as tolerated, to minimize the effects of the venom. The patient may need antibiotic coverage. Embedded particles can cause deep abscesses and will require wide radical debridement.

SHARKS, ALLIGATORS, AND WILD ANIMALS

It is possible to suffer injuries from such animals. Most often, it occurs because they are provoked or threatened in some fashion. The injuries can be severe with mangled extremity or even life-threatening injury with maceration and bleeding. They are treated in the same fashion as any other major trauma. Antibiotic coverage, tetanus toxoid injection, and cleansing the wound with copious saline solution, followed by debridement of devitalized tissue, are general standards.

KEY POINTS

Patients present with great agitation and fear following animal bites but may not recognize the seriousness of certain other stings that can cause greater damage to the body.

SECTION 11: General Care of Surgical Patient

73. Preoperative Rounds
74. Postoperative Care
75. Postsurgical Complications
76. Operative Care in General
77. Troubleshooting in the Operating Room
78. Bedside Procedures
79. Cancer Screening
80. What Test, What Method, What Instruments
81. Consultations and Ancillary Services
82. Surgical Challenge Situations
83. Wellness
84. Sign-out and Transfers
85. Safety in Surgery
86. Medical Malpractice Concerns

CHAPTER 73: Preoperative Rounds

INTRODUCTION

Checking the patient preoperatively is an extremely important step in preventing complications, reducing misunderstandings, conducting a smooth procedure, and avoiding medical malpractice suits. A busy surgeon walking in and starting an operation on a patient who has been draped is the worst professional conduct one can imagine. The preoperative checklist starts at the clinic when the surgeon first sees the patient and continues through multiple professionals until the incision is made.

EVALUATION AND MANAGEMENT

Preoperative assessment starts in the office or clinic itself. Is this patient a good risk to undergo the procedure? Is there an alternate way of treating the medical issue without surgery? What are the potential risks and complications? Should a less invasive procedure be chosen?

If the patient is a smoker, the patient should stop smoking for several weeks. If they are obese, effort should be made for weight reduction. If they are diabetic, blood sugar monitoring and dosage of medications need to be adjusted. Cardiac status should be assessed, especially on those who have prior cardiac history and on all older patients. If necessary, the patient should have a cardiology evaluation. Does the patient have a history of chronic obstructive pulmonary disease (COPD) or bronchial asthma? Do they need preoperative pulmonary therapy? What is the nutritional status? Do they have any chronic infections? What is the renal status? If there are any questions, further specialist evaluation is advised before scheduling elective surgery.

List of medications that the patient is taking is reviewed and followed up. Special attention is given to cardiac medications, antiplatelets, and anticoagulants they are on. If they are on any addictive habits with alcohol or drugs, risk of withdrawal symptoms is noted.

Routine preoperative tests include complete blood count, complete metabolic profile, urinalysis, electrocardiogram (ECG), and pregnancy test for women of childbearing age. Chest X-ray is done only if there are suspected cardiac or respiratory problems.

Making a preoperative check is an integral part of planning surgery. It can be in the form of rounds if the patient is already in the hospital or by previous day visits for preoperative instructions, with a review of chart if the patient is being admitted as an outpatient on the same day of surgery.

Either way, a second preoperative check should be conducted on the same day of surgery in the holding area, just prior to taking the patient to the operating room. Anesthesia should also do the same type of reviews ahead of time on the day of surgery, just prior to surgery.

It is extremely important to communicate with the patient and family members and answer all questions to their satisfaction. Often, the surgeon who examined the patient initially in the office or clinic may not remember all details offhand, and it is quite possible that another surgeon may be delegated to do the actual procedure. It is easy to classify a case as minor or routine and pass it down the chain of command. But to the patient, every intervention is scary and serious.

The first and foremost precaution is to avoid mistakes of operating on the wrong patient, wrong body part, wrong side, or do the wrong procedure. In spite of education and precautions, these "never ever" events do occur. A system should be established, and it must be followed rigorously which includes identification (ID) bands, asking the patient to identify themselves, asking them to recite their problems and the procedure they are planning to undergo, reviewing the chart for history, and a physical examination updated within last 48 hours. The surgeon who is going to do the procedure must physically examine the patient, review the chart, mark the incision site with marking ink, and discuss the case with the patient, anesthesiologist, and nurse.

A medical review should include coexisting medical conditions such as diabetes mellitus, hypertension, cardiac, pulmonary, renal, and bleeding disorders. Sometimes the patient complains of new onset symptoms of chest pain or asthma, which were not evident at the time of the initial office visit.

All medications that the patient is taking must be looked at, particularly for anticoagulants, antiplatelets, cardiac meds, insulin, etc.

The anticipated length of the operation and anticipated blood loss should be discussed with staff, and arrangements should be made for blood or blood products.

Any incidental infections such as skin infections and urinary or pulmonary infections must be looked at, and surgery must be postponed, if necessary.

Arrangements for preoperative or intraoperative antibiotic therapy must be made ahead of time.

All laboratory results must be available and carefully reviewed. Hemoglobin (Hb) and hematocrit (Hct) levels give information about anemia, conditions of chronic blood loss, and need for transfusion. Chemistry results of creatinine, blood urea nitrogen (BUN), sodium (Na), potassium (K), and chloride (Cl) are evaluated for chronic conditions. If necessary, ECG and chest X-ray are requested as well as blood gas analysis.

All imaging studies relevant to the case should be reviewed once again and made available in the operating room.

The anesthetic needs, intraoperative medications, positioning of the patient, and special requests must be discussed with the anesthesiologist before surgery.

Instructions on the need for instruments, suture materials, positioning of the patient on the table, type of surgery, nature of surgery, and key steps should be discussed with the nursing staff. Details of the actual procedure and steps of the case must be explained to the assistants who will be helping with the case.

Postoperative disposition such as admission, discharge, rehabilitation, or home health should be planned ahead of time.

KEY POINTS

Safety of the patient and avoiding errors are of paramount importance.

CHAPTER 74

Postoperative Care

INTRODUCTION

The surgeon's job does not end with performing the operation. It includes taking care of the patient after surgery, communicating with patient and family, and providing necessary follow-up. Many complications can arise related to surgery or anesthesia, and timely detection and attention can make a huge difference in the outcome. Unfortunately, we see many busy surgeons delegating postoperative care to assistants or residents and interns. For the patient, nothing can give more satisfaction than seeing the surgeon face-to-face during postoperative recovery.

EVALUATION AND MANAGEMENT

Postoperative care is just as important as preoperative and intraoperative care. Often, this is delegated to junior surgeons or assistants. The operative surgeon must supervise the postoperative care no matter how busy the person may be.

During the first 24 hours, attention is paid to vital signs, fluid balance, postanesthetic care, and cardiopulmonary and renal status. Concerns of postoperative bleeding following vascular, thoracic, cardiac, and such interventional procedures take priority. Is there development of hypotension, oliguria, bleeding from drain sites, or chest tubes? Is there any large hematoma formation following head and neck surgical procedures? Could there be intracranial bleeding or pericardial tamponade? Is there unexplained abdominal distension or abdominal compartment syndrome? Is the patient oversedated and comatose or undersedated and restless? Are the expected peripheral pulses palpable, or is there an occlusion of an artery or graft? Is there congestive heart failure or new onset neurological deficits? Is there a new collapse of lung or pneumothorax? Are there good adequate intravenous (IV) lines? Is the dressing getting saturated with blood too rapidly?

During the next 24 hours, attention is again paid to vital signs, intake and output, and cardiopulmonary and renal status. Antibiotic coverage is reviewed. Nutritional needs are addressed, and total parenteral nutrition (TPN) is started if prolonged starvation is anticipated. Ambulation and deep vein thrombosis (DVT) prophylaxis are addressed. Glycemic control, temperature control, and metabolic control are evaluated. Electrolytes, liver chemistries, and blood gases are analyzed.

Whenever possible, it is best to have all the team members, nursing staff, and other caregivers join for rounds together at a specified time every day for routine postoperative care. This would include checking the temperature chart, intake and output chart, laboratory values, physical examination, and wound care related to specific procedures. All the medications patient is receiving or not restarted from preoperative schedule are reviewed. Images are reviewed, and necessary new tests are ordered. Encouraging patient to take deep breaths, cough out and spit any phlegm, teaching incentive spirometry, and encouraging ambulation are part of recovery protocol. Wound dressing may need to be changed, and wounds may need to be inspected for dehiscence or infection. Drain sites and drainage amounts are checked. Specific surgery on specific organs is likely to have complications related to that procedure. For example, following thyroid surgery, one is to look out for hypocalcemia, hypothyroidism, thyroid storm, recurrent laryngeal nerve palsy, etc.

During the ensuing days, one would look for wound infections, wound care, anastomotic leaks, bowel functions, bowel sounds, pulmonary toilet, physiotherapy, and ambulation. One should remove each and every tube as soon as they are nonfunctional or unnecessary. Foley catheter and central lines are removed in a timely fashion. The patient should be extubated as soon as self-ventilation is possible. Antibiotics and pain medications are stopped in a timely fashion.

It is extremely important to communicate with the patient and family members as to the operative findings, current status, and future plans. Any and every complication should be treated immediately with corrective steps, and the family should be advised accordingly.

KEY POINTS

Success of the operation depends on careful follow-up during the postoperative period and timely correction of problems as they arise.

CHAPTER 75

Postsurgical Complications

INTRODUCTION

Complications do occur following surgery. It is the inherent nature. The only way to avoid complications is to not do surgery. However, one should do everything possible to minimize the complications. If they do occur, it is imperative to recognize them early on and take corrective steps so that it does not become worse. One should watch out and check the patient daily during the postoperative rounds.

SEROMA

Seroma is an accumulation of clear, thin fluid in the dissected tissue planes, usually lymphatic fluid, after axillary node dissection, mastectomy, groin node dissection, or ventral hernia repair. It is a soft swelling with fluctuation. The fluid can be aspirated with a sterile technique and compression dressing applied. Over a period of time, they usually resolve spontaneously.

HEMATOMA

Hematoma is bleeding into the tissues from small arteries or due to coagulation disorders. It is a firm, solid swelling with no fluctuation. They are seen after scrotal or testicular surgery, head and neck surgery, or vascular procedures. They can occur internally and cause unexplained postoperative anemia. Prevention at surgery includes meticulous hemostasis, correction of coagulation abnormalities, use of topical hemostatic agents such as Avitene™ or Surgicel®, use of drains in cavities and large wounds, and compression bandages. Small hematomas can resolve. Larger ones are best evacuated, irrigated, and drained in the operating room.

WOUND INFECTION

Most of them are preventable by improving attention to detail on techniques and sterility. Prophylactic antibiotics are useful. If wound infection is anticipated from a contaminated case, the wound can be partially left open. Once a wound infection is recognized by the clinical appearance of redness, wound drainage, or fever, the infected wound needs to be cleaned adequately to drain the fluid. The wound is opened by removing the skin sutures. Cultures are taken, and appropriate antibiotics are given. Daily wound care with irrigation and dressings is provided.

ABDOMINAL WOUND DEHISCENCE

Burst abdomen and evisceration can occur due to rupture of a full-depth wound. It usually occurs 7-10 days after surgery. The causes could be due to technical errors, type of suture materials, tense abdomen, excess tension, deep infections, hematoma, immunocompromised status, and nutritional deficiencies. A telltale sign is frequent drainage of a pinkish fluid seeping from the wound with bogginess. Upon suspicion, the best option is to take the patient to the operating room and explore the wound under sterile conditions. If there is evidence of dehiscence, the wound is closed with multiple retention sutures, drained, and an abdominal binder applied.

POSTOPERATIVE FEVER

Common causes are pulmonary atelectasis, surgical site infection, urinary infection, intravenous (IV) site phlebitis, line-related infections, and deep-seated or intra-abdominal infections. Numerous other possibilities do exist since fever is a reaction of the body to a challenge. Antipyretic medications, cooling blankets, or tepid sponge baths do help. More important is to find the cause of fever and address the same. This may involve attention to pulmonary hygiene, removal of unwanted lines, changing antibiotics, and checking for wound infections.

DEEP VEIN THROMBOSIS AND PULMONARY EMBOLISM

Deep vein thrombosis (DVT) prophylaxis is now observed as a mandatory protocol in many hospitals. All patients should be ambulated as soon as possible. Those who are nonambulatory for >24 hours should receive DVT prophylaxis. This includes the use of elastic stocking, sequential compression devices, and low-dose anticoagulants using mini-dose heparin, Fragmin®, or Arixtra®.

Patients should be examined for calf tenderness on a daily basis, and if any swelling or pain is noted, they should be evaluated further with a venous sonogram. As soon as DVT is confirmed, IV or oral medications for a full anticoagulation protocol are started. If anticoagulation is contraindicated for any reason, then consideration is given for a vena caval filter placement. Diagnosis of pulmonary embolism (PE) is confirmed by a computed tomography (CT) angiogram of pulmonary veins. If PE is confirmed, in addition to anticoagulation and systemic cardiovascular support, consideration is given for focused thrombolytic therapy into the clot using a transcatheter method.

PROLONGED PARALYTIC ILEUS

Following abdominal surgery or after major insults to the body, ileus or lack of peristalsis is noted to occur. The precise mechanism is poorly understood. However, certain factors such as prolonged open surgery, peritonitis, infections, bleeding, contamination, and excessive manipulation contribute to more ileus, as compared to laparoscopic procedures, quick procedures, and clean cases. Certain drugs, such as opioids and psychotropics, can also cause ileus, as well as pneumonia and electrolyte abnormalities. The abdomen is distended and silent with absent bowel sounds. It is important to recognize early postoperative bowel obstruction, anastomotic problems, and intra-abdominal sepsis from ileus. If the ileus does not resolve in 1 week, a CT scan or contrast studies are done to rule out mechanical problems. Medications such as IV Reglan or rectal suppositories might help. Usually, the ileus clears up spontaneously.

ATELECTASIS AND PNEUMONIA

Postoperative pulmonary problems, especially following general anesthesia and abdominal surgery, need attention. Secretions accumulate, peripheral alveoli remain unexpanded, and secondary infection and pneumonia set in, leading to respiratory insufficiency. Smoking, obesity, emphysema, endotracheal intubation, prolonged surgery, ventilator dependency, aspiration, pain due to abdominal surgery, and nasogastric (NG) tube are contributing factors. Patients are asked to take deep breaths and cough, ambulated as soon as possible, the NG tube is removed as soon as possible, incentive spirometry device is given, and if necessary, nasotracheal suctioning is done. In more serious cases, an X-ray is done, and bronchoscopic aspiration is done.

ABDOMINAL COMPARTMENT SYNDROME

This is a rare but well-established postoperative complication that can happen following major surgery, acute pancreatitis, trauma, or shock followed by aggressive fluid resuscitation, sepsis, and cardiogenic shock. There is marked edema and capillary leak resulting in tenseness and distension of the abdomen. There is increased bladder pressure and abdominal pressure, leading to decreased venous return, hypotension, and further oliguria. Diagnosis is by clinical suspicion and measurement of bladder pressure. Bladder pressure is measured with an indwelling Foley catheter connected to a simple water manometer. Bladder pressure of >30 cm of water is suggestive of abdominal compartment syndrome. The abdomen is opened at the bedside in the intensive care unit (ICU) or in the operative room, bowels are allowed to expand out, and the wound is covered in a suitable fashion with wet towels or plastic material for secondary closure at a later date.

CARDIAC PROBLEMS

Many of the older patients and those with prior cardiac problems can easily go into variety of postsurgical cardiac problems. Most common is cardiac arrhythmia of varying nature. Continuous electrocardiogram (ECG) monitoring is usually provided in the immediate postoperative period. They can go into congestive heart failure or even acute myocardial infarction since surgery is a stress, and fluid management can be fluctuant for a certain period of time. Cardiology consultation and appropriate management will be needed.

RENAL AND URINARY PROBLEMS

Common problems are urinary retention and inability to void, especially in men related to pain, prostate enlargement, and sedation. They may need catheterization. It is better to leave an indwelling Foley catheter for 2 or 3 days. Another commonly noted issue would be low urine output.

This could be due to hypovolemia or renal insult secondary to sepsis or shock. Initially, fluid challenge is given. If there is no improvement, low-dose diuretics are given. Urinary tract infections are easy to set in during postsurgical period.

GLYCEMIC CONTROL

Diabetic patients can develop fluctuating levels of blood sugar, more often hyperglycemia than hypoglycemia. Patients will not be taking their usual medications and following their dietary regulations. Intravenous fluid and total parenteral nutrition (TPN), along with postsurgical stress, can further complicate the glucose regulation. Frequent blood sugar monitoring and continuous infusion of insulin may be required.

NEUROLOGICAL PROBLEMS

Patients can go into delirium tremens, psychosis, cognitive disorders, seizures, and withdrawal symptoms. They could have been on alcohol or addictive drugs preoperatively. It can also be due to surgery and anesthesia. They could be having preexisting neurological problems. Surgery and anesthesia can aggravate their mental status. They will need appropriate medications, close observation, and safety measures to prevent falls, agitation, and involuntary removal of catheters and tubes.

KEY POINTS

Many postoperative complications can arise. The surgeon has to be on the lookout to identify them and correct them early on.

CHAPTER 76

Operative Care in General

INTRODUCTION

Performing surgery is a privilege and honor and should not be considered a chore. A certain amount of discipline and decorum is to be observed as if entering a temple of worship. It is for the safety of the patient and for efficient functioning of the operating room. Sterile precautions are to be observed by everyone. Punctuality is to be maintained. Unnecessary disturbances, small talk, and cell phone conversations are to be minimized. The focus should be on patient care and patient safety.

MANAGEMENT

To the surgeon, the operating room is the temple of worship or God's workshop. If God created us, then repair of God's creations is a service to God. Entering and working in this place should be seen as a privilege and honor. The work here should not be seen as a chore by any one of the healthcare providers. It requires teamwork to do the highest level of service.

One should be mentally and physically prepared to enter the operating room. It is not a place for casual conversations or gatherings. A certain amount of discipline, decorum, and dignity is to be observed at every level.

Scrub suits, hats, eye protection, and masks are to be worn by everyone when entering the sterile areas to reduce contamination and protect the patient. There has been much discussion in the literature as to the need for scrub suits and types of hats. It is better to wear them instead of doing surgery in street clothes and gowns. Type of shoes should be ones used exclusively in the operating room and ergonomically comfortable. Shoe covers are desirable again to reduce spillage of body fluids.

Cell phones, social media, loud music, and casual conversations are to be minimized to reduce distractions.

Scrubbing, gloving, and gowning are to be observed carefully to enhance maximum sterility.

The operating crew should wash and cleanse the table, linens, and floor and prepare the room with attention to detail after every case. The nurses should be cautious about sterilizing the instruments and keeping them ready for each case.

The surgeon, anesthesiologist, and nurses should go over each case just before taking the patient to the operating room and have communication on the type of surgery, instruments needed, imaging studies reviewed, expected blood loss or complication, and any other special needs during or after the operation. Consent and chart are rechecked.

Skin preparation includes clipping the hair, washing the operative field with antiseptics, and draping with sterile towels and sheets. Different types of skin preparations have been described. Generally, chlorhexidine or betadine is used for initial washing and painting the field, followed by alcohol swab of the incision line.

Lighting should be adjusted, cautery machine and suction machine checked, and anesthesia administered appropriately. Smoke evacuators, energy equipment, cameras, and laparoscopic setups are verified.

Before the knife is handed to the surgeon, a final "time out" is observed. All members in the operating room should participate in this ritual when the patient identification (ID) is verified, consent is read, side and site of surgery are reaffirmed, type and nature of surgery are repeated, nurses verify that all instruments are available, anesthesiologist verifies that necessary medications and antibiotics have been administered, and all members agree that all systems are a "go."

During surgery, it is important for the surgeon to minimize the operating time without compromising on quality of care. This is not to hurry up and do a rush job. This can be achieved by avoiding unnecessary dissections, knowing the exact anatomy, getting hemostasis at every level before going into the next step, understanding the planes of dissection, focusing on the procedure that was planned, and having constant communication with the assistant and scrub nurse as to what to expect at each step. If everything is done purposefully, carefully, and meticulously, one will save a lot of time and aggravation in the end.

KEY POINTS

Surgery is an art and a science. It is like an opera and music. If all parties do their part in a smooth and coordinated fashion, the end result is pleasant.

CHAPTER 77

Troubleshooting in the Operating Room

INTRODUCTION

Surgeons are at times called to help with problems noted by other surgeons or other specialists. Sometimes it is the surgeon's own complication that needs troubleshooting. Handling the crisis in an effective manner is what makes the surgeon more respectful. It comes with experience but also needs confidence, clinical knowledge, and technical skill. An unexpected turn of events may arise due to injury to organs other than the surgery site, excessive bleeding, inability to complete the procedure, and need for technical help.

EVALUATION AND MANAGEMENT

During surgery, many unforeseen events can occur. It may be out of your control, complications caused by others, or your own complications. Handling these crisis situations in an efficient manner needs patience, a calm demeanor, competence, and knowledge.

Sometimes, we get phone calls from obstetrics and gynecologists, urologists, and junior surgeons as they have encountered problems during the procedure. They may have noticed too many adhesions between bowels, injured the bowel or urinary bladder, or excessive bleeding is encountered.

As I arrive at the scene, I advise them to apply packing and hold everything until I scrub in and evaluate the situation by myself.

One common problem I often notice is that they are working through a small incision with difficult exposure. I do not hesitate to extend the incision to get proper exposure.

Next, I focus on the area of problem by packing away the rest of the abdomen and applying proper retractors and lighting. Then I evaluate the injury or pathology and decide on the corrective step.

Adhesions between bowel loops and other structures preventing exposure of pelvis is a common problem noted by gynecologists. Find an easily mobile and free spot and work slowly forward. Flip the bowel from one side to the other and work a little from each side. Tiny snips with sharp scissors, along with right amount of stretching in either direction, will facilitate slow but steady progress. Do not cut anything blindly. A good deal of finger dissection and separation will go a long way. Irrigating the area with small amounts of saline will soften the area and make the dissection easier. If a certain spot appears very difficult and densely adherent, leave that spot for a while, and go to another spot that allows easier separation. Eventually, they will meet and allow completion.

Bowel injuries of fresh nature under sterile conditions can be repaired primarily during an operation. Make sure that the devitalized edges are trimmed and a proper two-layer closure is done securely. It would be necessary to lyse any adhesions that are present at the area in order to get a good repair.

Urinary bladder injuries can also be repaired in two layers. Always use absorbable suture materials. An indwelling Foley catheter is placed, bladder is filled with sterile irrigation solution, and the site of injury can be rechecked for leak. If there is any question, the pelvis is drained with a closed suction drainage system.

Injury to the bile duct occurs more often after advent of laparoscopic cholecystectomy. Corrective repair depends on the location and extent of damage. Ideal step is to convert the procedure to open and assess the damage precisely. A cystic duct cholangiogram is done to visualize the entire biliary tree in which one should see the bifurcation, all the branches and the entire common bile duct with flow of dye into the duodenum. If the surgeon is not experienced or comfortable, the best step is to complete the cholecystectomy, drain the area, and transfer patient to a tertiary care center immediately. If the damage is extensive, one may need a more complex Roux-en-Y anastomosis to jejunum. Fresh clean-cut injury to a single spot on the common bile duct can be primarily repaired, with or without a T-tube drainage of the bile duct. Subhepatic space is drained with closed suction drainage system after making sure good hemostasis has been achieved.

Injury to the ureter can be repaired primarily over a ureteric stent with drainage of the area. In order to avoid tension, the ureter or kidney may have to be mobilized from its bed. The cut ends are fish-mouthed for a wider anastomosis. If energy devices, such as harmonic scalpel, were used during the injury, the cut ends would have coagulated capillaries, and primary closure will not heal properly. A segment of the ureter may have to be excised to get clean bleeding healthy edges. Further repair will need help of a qualified urologist.

Excessive bleeding can be controlled once the area of bleeding is identified. Most arterial and venous injuries can be closed with fine sutures. At the conclusion of arterial repair, one should make sure distal pulses are palpable. Anticoagulation with heparin is given when the artery is clamped.

All repairs or anastomosis follow similar principles. There should be no tension at the suture lines. The edges should be viable and pink with good vascularity. There should be no disease at the area of suturing. The suturing should be technically sound and watertight.

After the immediate problem is resolved, I usually depart, allowing the original team to complete the operation. It is important to avoid making any critical or derogatory comments.

KEY POINTS

Various technical and logistic problems can arise during surgery. They need to be addressed without getting perturbed.

Bedside Procedures

INTRODUCTION

Surgeons are asked to perform many bedside procedures, either because it is time-consuming to transfer the patient to the operating room or it poses a risk to do so. Moreover, it is cost-saving and feasible to do the procedure without a major risk to the patient. Some such procedures are insertion of central venous pressure line, cut down for venous access, tracheostomy, gastroscopy, colonoscopy, insertion of percutaneous endoscopic gastrostomy (PEG tube placement), incision and drainage of abscesses, and debridement of wounds.

INSERTION OF CENTRAL LINE

Often a central line (**Fig. 78.1**) placement is very helpful in patient management in situations such as:
- The patient is in shock and needs a reliable intravenous (IV) route for administration of fluids and medications.
- There are no peripheral veins available in a patient who needs IV fluids and medicines.
- The patient needs central venous pressure monitoring to know the filling pressure.
- The patient is undergoing major surgery, and blood transfusion and IV fluids are to be administered rapidly.
- The central line has three lumens, and they can be used for different purposes instead of finding multiple IV sites.
- Administration of concentrated solutions such as total parenteral nutrition (TPN) with 20% glucose
- Extravasation of certain medications can cause severe chemical burns and must be administered into a central vein.

The central line can be inserted by jugular, subclavian, or femoral vein approaches.

JUGULAR APPROACH

Place the patient in head down position (Trendelenburg position) by tilting the bed. Place a rolled towel under the shoulder to lift up the clavicles. The landmarks are anterior border of the sternomastoid muscle, suprasternal notch, and mandibular margin. Feel for the carotid artery. Turn the face away from the side of insertion. Find the area of division of the two heads of sternomastoid insertion. In anterior approach, the needle puncture will be at the bifurcation of the two heads of the muscle. In the posterior approach, the needle puncture will be at the mid-part of the posterior edge of the muscle. Inject a small amount of lidocaine. Use a small-size needle with small size guidewire first (micropuncture kit). First, advance the needle with a syringe to tap into the vein, and once blood is drawn, remove the syringe and insert the guidewire through the needle. Then make a small incision at the entrance of the puncture point on the skin, enough to advance a dilator over the guidewire. Then replace the smaller guidewire with a larger guidewire and dilator. Finally, advance the triple-lumen central line over the larger guidewire. Aspirate blood, flush with heparin solution, and suture the line securely to skin. Apply an Opsite dressing over the insertion site. Take a chest X-ray and review it to make sure that the line is in good position and there is no pneumothorax or hemothorax. Make sure the fluid is flowing properly.

SUBCLAVIAN APPROACH

The positioning of the patient is the same as above. The landmarks are suprasternal notch and mid-point of the inferior border of clavicle. The needle is advanced slowly toward the neck from the inferior border of center of clavicle. Once blood is aspirated, the guidewire is advanced, and the procedure is completed as above.

FEMORAL APPROACH

The patient is in supine position with the thighs slightly abducted. Feel the femoral artery, pubic tuberosity, and anterior superior iliac spine. The femoral vein will be

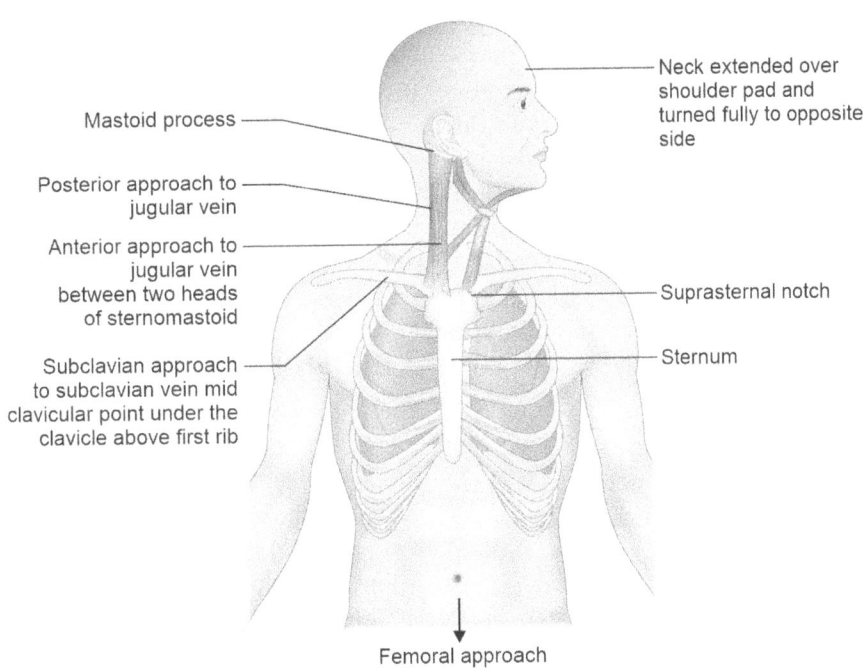

Fig. 78.1: Insertions of central line.

just medial to the femoral artery, just below the inguinal ligament in the mid-inguinal region. The needle is advanced downward with a slight tilt toward the pelvis. Once blood is aspirated, advance the guidewire and complete the procedure as above.

CUT DOWN FOR INTRAVENOUS ACCESS

Sometimes, it will be necessary to do a cut down to get an intravenous (IV) access. This is often needed in children and infants. Sometimes, there is a dire need to infuse large amounts of blood rapidly, and the central line may not be accessible. The first option is to cut down at the groin via long saphenous vein. Feel the femoral artery, mid-inguinal point between pubic tuberosity, and anterior superior iliac spine. The long saphenous vein is usually located 1 inch below and medial to the femoral artery pulsation at the mid-inguinal point. Make a transverse incision and dissect the fat and subcutaneous tissue. Isolate one inch length of the saphenous vein. Make the cut down between two loops of silk. In adults, the whole IV tubing can be threaded into it and advanced into the femoral or iliac vein. In children, an angiocath no. 18 size can be advanced. Securely suture the catheter to the skin, close the wound, and apply a dressing.

ENDOTRACHEAL INTUBATION

Emergency airway management is a life-saving measure, and physicians should be familiar with the technique. First, inspect the oral cavity, open up the jaws, set up the laryngoscope and suction device, select the appropriate size endotracheal tube, and have help stand by. Keep a rolled towel under the shoulder to keep the neck extended. Extend the neck as far as possible, open the mouth as wide as possible, and insert the blade of the laryngoscope deep at the base of the tongue. Forcibly lift the base of the tongue to expose the uvula and the laryngeal opening underneath. Insert the endotracheal tube into the laryngeal opening, inflate the balloon, connect the Ambu® bag, and give breathings. Check for equal breath sounds on both sides using the stethoscope with the ventilation, check over the epigastrium to make sure there is no gastric insufflation, and verify the carbon dioxide (CO_2) monitor and oxygen (O_2) saturation to ensure proper ventilation and oxygenation. Then tape it down securely with a bite block next to the endotracheal tube.

TRACHEOSTOMY

Keep the neck extended over a shoulder pad. Prep and drape the front of the neck. Inject local anesthesia over the front of the neck for 2 inches in length from cricoid cartilage down. Make a vertical incision over this same length starting from cricoid cartilage. Split the strap muscles to expose the thyroid fascia. Divide the isthmus of thyroid between clamps to expose the tracheal rings. Clear the second, third, and fourth rings of trachea for tracheotomy. Keep the tracheostomy tube ready, check the balloon, and keep it lightly lubricated with the trocar inside the outer tube. Make a cruciate incision over the second ring; insert a hemostat or tracheal dilator to widen the opening in the trachea large enough to insert the tracheostomy tube. Insert the tracheostomy tube into the tracheal lumen simultaneously as one withdraws the endotracheal tube if one is present. Insert the tracheostomy tube, remove the trocar, insert the inner tube, connect the Ambu® bag, and oxygen and ventilate. Securely ligate the tracheostomy tube around the neck and apply a light dressing. Suture the edges of the wound if necessary. Check for equal breath sounds on both lung fields and obtain a chest X-ray to check lung condition.

DEBRIDEMENT OF WOUND

Surgeons are very often called in to debride necrotic wounds. This may be the result of a decubitus ulcer, necrotizing fasciitis, diabetic gangrene, or infected injuries. Unless the necrotic and nonviable tissues are sharply excised, the wounds do not granulate well, and bacterial infection continues to harbor in the depths.

Using sterile instruments and gloved hands, the debridement is started on the surface and slowly carried to deeper levels. Nonviable tissues are painless since they are dead tissues; however, the deeper tissues may be sensitive. Hence, either a sedation or analgesic is given before touching deeper tissues. Sometimes it may be necessary to give a general anesthesia and do this in the operating room. All tissues in the base of the debrided wound should be pink or bleeding. One may encounter excessive bleeding or spurting spots. With compression, some of them may stop, otherwise, suture ligation or cauterization of the spot will be necessary. Cultures of the deep tissues are always taken to adjust the antibiotic coverage. Covering of the debrided open wound is done initially with wet saline gauze and compression dressing.

Afterward, a moisturizing cream-like hydrogel is applied to the wound base. It is better to avoid betadine or other antiseptics to the wound base.

INCISION AND DRAINAGE OF ABSCESS

This may sound like a simple procedure, especially when there is a superficial abscess pointing and ready to rupture. The patient will be willing to have it drained because of the pain; however, it requires a certain amount of precaution. Injecting local anesthesia may be difficult due to the inflammation over it. IV sedation or analgesic is required. A small puncture or incision will allow some of the pus to be drained, but it may not resolve completely. An adequate-length incision must be made, and the necrotic tissue inside must be completely evacuated. Many of the skin abscesses may have an infected sebaceous cyst as the causative factor. They may have cheesy and pultaceous material inside, requiring manual evacuation. Another scenario is a carbuncle, which has multiple purulent spots on the surface of a thick inflamed cellulitis area. This will require a wide incision and deep debridement under anesthesia since it is not one single abscess cavity. There is infection and necrosis deep under the skin, which will become necrotic if left alone.

BEDSIDE LAPAROTOMY

There are occasions when a bedside laparotomy is required. It could be because patient is attached to too many life support devices or because the regular operating room is not available for an emergency. One such situation is abdominal compartment syndrome. Blood pressure is low, urine out is low, and abdomen is tense with high bladder pressure. Under sterile precautions, vertical laparotomy incision is made. As soon as peritoneal cavity is opened, the bowels bulge out. Drains are placed inside the abdomen, and it is covered with wet towels and a plastic silo. Another situation is for a second look laparotomy for patients already treated for mesenteric ischemia.

OTHER PROCEDURES

In addition to the above several other bedside procedures are done. Some of them include bronchoscopy, percutaneous tracheostomy, placement of Swan Ganz catheter, placement of temporary dialysis catheters, placement of temporary pacemakers, upper and lower gastrointestinal (GI) endoscopies, percutaneous gastrostomy, placement of chest tubes, and placement of arterial lines, to name a few.

GENERAL PRECAUTIONS

Bedside procedures need the same caution and protocols as regular operating room procedures. Consent should be documented, and "time out" should be observed. Operating staff and assisting personnel should wear sterile gowns, mask and hat, and should scrub and wear gloves. Proper lighting and instruments are needed. The operation site should be prepped and draped as usual and sterile precautions should be observed.

KEY POINTS

Several procedures can be done at the bedside with sterile precautions and by observing safety measures. It is more convenient for the patient and caregivers. It is also more cost-effective.

CHAPTER 79

Cancer Screening

INTRODUCTION

Early detection of cancer has a better chance of cure. This is well proven in breast cancers, colorectal cancers, and skin cancers. Some of the cancers can probably be prevented from occurring by taking precautionary measures. For example, colonoscopy and removal of polyps can reduce incidence of colorectal cancers; use of sunscreens and avoiding exposure to the sun can reduce melanoma of skin. Lifestyle habits such as diet, exercise, and avoidance of alcohol or smoking can reduce various malignancies. Screening for cancer and having regular medical checkups are good health measures.

"I want to know if I have a cancer." Patients want this information often. Physicians are also supposed to do cancer screenings to diagnose and treat cancers early for a better outcome.

There is no single test for finding cancers. However, there are several steps one can take in preventative healthcare.

SKIN

Early diagnosis of melanoma and squamous cell cancers can lead to curative treatments by simple wide local excisions. Once they are advanced, cure rates go down even after complex therapies. Patients and physicians are advised to have any and every abnormal looking skin lesion examined, biopsied, or excised if necessary.

Protecting against sun exposure is a useful measure. One may avoid direct exposure to the sun, apply sunscreen lotion, or cover up the body with clothing when outside.

BREAST

Early diagnosis gives an almost 90% chance for a permanent cure. Routine physical examination, self-examination, and screening mammograms are the available tools. Those who have a family history of breast cancers or who had prior gynecological (GYN) cancers are at a higher risk. Gene testing for *BRCA* gene mutations can be done for those at high risk.

CERVIX

Routine pap smears and regular GYN checkups are useful tools. Abnormal menstrual cycles or flows are investigated.

Human papilloma virus (HPV) vaccine on a prophylactic basis has been found very effective in preventing carcinoma of cervix. As a result, the incidence of cancer of cervix has markedly decreased in advanced countries. In addition, HPV vaccine is found to reduce incidence of cancer of penis, throat, tongue, and tonsils.

LUNG

Avoid smoking habits at all costs. Also, avoid pollution if possible, whether it is work related or environment related. Those who have history of smoking for 30 years or quit smoking within the past 15 years, and between age group 55 and 80 are recommended to have one low-dose computed tomography (LDCT) scan of chest every year. Obtain physical examination and tests upon noticing coughing spells or hemoptysis.

COLORECTAL

Report any change in bowel habits or rectal bleeding for further evaluation. Routine screening of the stool for microscopic blood by hemoccult testing is a good first step. Other tests of value are the fecal immunoassay test (FIT) for colonic blood and the Cologuard test, which uses deoxyribonucleic acid (DNA) analysis of the stool for early cancers and polyps. A blood test for screening is also in the developmental stage. A screening colonoscopy once every 10 years is recommended. Polyps diagnosed early can be removed by the endoscope, thus preventing cancer formation.

PROSTATE

A routine prostate-specific antigen (PSA) has certain advantages. A routine rectal examination and prostate ultrasound can be done to pick up occult lesions.

LUMPS AND BUMPS

All abnormal lumps and bumps should be evaluated. They could be enlarged lymph nodes, which could, in turn, be spread from another source or a primary lymphoma.

TESTICULAR

Routine physical examinations should include palpation of testes for tumors, hydrocele, and hernia. Patients are also to report any abnormalities.

VISCERAL MALIGNANCIES

One must follow up on unexplained weight loss, loss of appetite, vomiting, abdominal pain, or vomiting blood. A complete physical examination and necessary tests that may include a CT scan or gastrointestinal (GI) endoscopy are recommended.

LIVER CANCERS

Vaccination against hepatitis A and B has reduced incidence of hepatoma. Avoidance of hepatitis C by taking precautions against needle punctures and needle sharing and reduction of alcohol addiction have also reduced liver cancers.

BRAIN TUMORS

Do not ignore unusual headaches, visual or hearing disturbances, falls, blackouts, fainting spells, or balancing problems. Consult a neurologist and obtain a CT scan or magnetic resonance imaging (MRI) of the brain.

BLOOD TEST

A regular complete blood count with peripheral smear can reveal leukemia, anemia, and bone marrow abnormalities.

Certain markers for cancers such as C-reactive protein (CRP), alpha-fetoproteins, CA-19, and CA-125 have been described but are not specific for diagnosis. Newer efforts to find a genetic abnormality for cancer are being worked on.

Blood tests to find different cancers are being developed and are called "liquid biopsy." Circulating cancer DNA particles can be detected for early diagnosis in several situations.

OTHER STEPS

Exercise regularly, eat a healthy diet, avoid addiction to alcohol, avoid smoking and drugs, and live in a healthy neighborhood.

A routine physical examination by a primary care physician and routine tests to evaluate any unusual symptoms are recommended.

KEY POINTS

It behooves both patients and physicians to undertake preventive measures and diagnostic efforts to detect cancers early. It is good health care. Early treatments of cancers have a better chance of a cure.

CHAPTER 80

What Test, What Method, What Instruments

INTRODUCTION

When choosing a type of test or a type of operation, the physician should recommend the best for the patient, not only from financial point but also from medical point. Several tests and options of therapy with different protocols using different instruments are available with the aim of reaching the same goal.

DISCUSSION

With advancing technology and progress in healthcare science, a wide array of choices is available to the physicians to make the diagnosis, confirm it, and then treat it. Cost of health care is a concern to all. Patients may demand the cutting-edge technology they had heard from marketing strategies of the hospital or from social media and advertisements. It is prudent for the physician to make the quickest diagnosis with least expenses and provide the best treatment under given circumstances. However, it is not uncommon to lose sight during marketing, competition, and income concerns. Multiple tests are often performed giving the same information and can be avoided.

For general diagnostic tests, one has availability of ultrasound, computed tomography (CT) scan, or magnetic resonance imaging (MRI) scan. Ultrasound is considered a poor man's CT scan since the cost is one-tenth and a good deal of information can be gathered. Portable and bedside quick tests can be performed with ultrasound technology. Diagnoses of gallbladder stones or kidney problems or stones, urinary bladder problems, tubo-ovarian or uterine problems, pregnancy-related issues, deep vein thrombosis, carotid artery screening, abdominal aortic aneurysm screening and peripheral vascular screening, pericardial effusion, abdominal trauma [focused assessment with sonography for trauma (FAST)], breast masses and thyroid masses, torsion of testicle, hydrocele are instances where ultrasound technology is superior.

The CT scan is superior for intracranial lesions and head trauma, mediastinal pathology, and certain abdominal conditions. Acute appendicitis can be accurately diagnosed 95% of the times by CT scan. However, not all cases of suspected appendicitis need a CT scan, if diagnosis is obvious by clinical means. It is also superior in evaluating intra-abdominal malignancies, particularly pancreatic cancers, metastatic deposits in liver, splenic conditions, diaphragmatic conditions, abdominal aortic aneurysms, retroperitoneal lesions, and pelvic pathologies.

The MRI scan is superior in evaluating joint conditions, spinal cord or vertebral problems, and intracranial problems. Magnetic resonance cholangiopancreatography (MRCP) is an excellent noninvasive alternative to doing endoscopic retrograde cholangiopancreatography (ERCP). Magnetic resonance angiogram (MRA) is useful as an outpatient procedure that does not involve injection of contrast material for evaluation of blood vessels.

When it comes to doing surgery, the time-honored and gold standard is open incision surgery. It is still the best way for all pathologies involving the skin and subcutaneous tissues.

Abdominal wall procedures, particularly inguinal hernia and incisional hernia repairs, have seen major changes in the recent past. What was done by open incision surgery became laparoscopic procedure, and now it is becoming robotic-assisted surgery. The advantage claimed for laparoscopic and robotic approaches is that the incisions are small, and hence the postoperative pain is less and return to work is faster. However, the costs are exponentially high and new sets of complications, some of which are life-threatening, can occur. Hernia in childhood and small umbilical hernia are easily repaired with a small skin incision. Very large inguinoscrotal hernia requires proper open surgery to dissect out the bowel. Setup for robotics is time-consuming and often risky in emergency situations such as strangulated or incarcerated hernia. Proper familiarity with the instruments, setup requirements, and comfort level of surgeon and assisting staff are important factors. In most poor countries, open inguinal hernia repair is the only option since the hospitals cannot afford to buy expensive hardware and disposable components.

For elective intra-abdominal procedures, laparoscopic method has become a preferred option in many instances, particularly for elective cholecystectomy and appendectomy. Sometimes laparoscopic-assisted hybrid procedures are done to reduce the size of open incisions and reduce the open exposure time of abdominal viscera. Different energy devices, stapling devices, tackers, and clips are used to facilitate these steps. It is prudent for the surgeon to be completely familiar with these devices, which are excellent but can also sometimes cause their own complications.

Robotic surgery is most useful in fine dissections and separation of tissues with minimal trauma to surrounding tissues and for accuracy of dissection and suture placements. They are often useful in doing radical prostatectomy for cancer of prostate, with minimal damage to surrounding nerves and blood vessels to retain continence and sexual functions. Other uses are in gynecological malignancies for pelvic and retroperitoneal lymph node dissections. Robotics are finding uses in many other types of surgery. However, it is not clear if they are really needed for many such operations, even though robotics are steadily gaining popularity with added benefits of better ergonomics, magnification, and artificial intelligence.

Several operations and instruments are introduced as new and better, but only to be abandoned after a while. For example, lasers were introduced initially for cholecystectomy as the key item for minimally invasive surgery. Lasers were subsequently abandoned for this procedure since laparoscopy was the key item and energy source could be just electrocautery. Lap-bands were introduced for obesity management, but they were abandoned due to various complications. Surgeon needs to be constantly vigilant. Learning is a life-long process.

Innovative methods of doing minimally invasive surgery touting smaller or nonvisible incisions have been introduced. Such procedures include natural orifice transluminal endoscopic surgery (NOTES) to remove organs such as gallbladder and appendix through natural orifices such as vaginal cuff or through the stomach, or transrectal endoscopic microsurgery (TEM) for removal of rectal tumors, and single incision laparoscopic surgery (SILS) where all the instruments for laparoscopic surgery are introduced through a single incision for cholecystectomy or appendectomy. However, these procedures are more difficult, with more complications and require special training and instruments. They are not for everyday practice by average surgeon. Safety of the patient is more important than adventurism.

KEY POINTS

Surgeon should choose the type of approach based on safety and benefit for the patient, and the surgeon should be experienced and comfortable with the use of the special instruments and equipment. Whatever method is safe in the surgeon's hands is the best method.

CHAPTER 81

Consultations and Ancillary Services

INTRODUCTION

Surgery is a teamwork and often requires participation from multiple specialists. Requesting for support and help from such specialists is prudent and good practice. Part of decision-making in surgery is to know when to ask for help and what type of support can be expected from other specialists in managing the patient.

DISCUSSION

Modern medicine mandates multiple specialists working together for the common cause of patient wellness. It is not possible for a general surgeon to manage all the cases independently anymore. Requesting appropriate consultations in a timely fashion allows better patient outcome. The surgeon can save time and focus on the operative procedure in the process.

Interventional radiologists can provide great help in multiple ways. Intra-abdominal abscesses such as appendiceal abscess, diverticular abscess, subphrenic abscess, and pelvic abscess can be drained percutaneously with computed tomography (CT) guidance and progress followed with further CT scans. This has reduced the need for open surgery in presence of pus and infections, with associated wound infections.

Cholecystostomy tube placement for acalculous cholecystitis is useful in acutely ill patients. Subsequent definitive surgery, if necessary, can be planned with less contamination and with better health of the patient.

Another scenario is management of gastrointestinal (GI) bleeding, when a selective angiogram can pinpoint the area of bleeding and selective embolization of the artery can stop the bleeding.

They can insert peripherally inserted central lines, dialysis catheters, and infusaports. They can do peripheral angiograms and participate in endovascular procedures and give thrombolytic therapy for emboli, thus reducing the need for open surgery under emergency conditions.

Placement of stents for portal hypertension [transjugular intrahepatic portosystemic shunt (TIPS)] has reduced the need for complex portosystemic shunts.

Selective angiogram and embolization of bleeding vessels are valuable in pelvic fractures, hemobilia, and head and neck trauma.

Breast radiologists can perform percutaneous diagnostic biopsies and place markers at the biopsy site for further management.

Many CT-guided biopsies of internal tissues have reduced the need for open biopsy and further surgery in certain situations.

Gastroenterologists can be of great help in diagnosing and treating a variety of GI surgical problems. Endoscopy helps with diagnosing various intraluminal lesions, both visually and by biopsy. GI bleeding sites can be located and often treated by endoscopic method. Inflammatory bowel diseases are comanaged with them. Placement of percutaneous feeding gastrostomy with upper endoscopy (PEG tube) is useful in bedridden and critically ill patients. Endoscopic ultrasounds can help with staging of cancers.

Other specialists are consulted according to the need, such as infectious diseases consultant for septic conditions, intensive care consultant for patients with multiple organ failures, cardiologist, pulmonologist, nephrologist, anesthesiologist, and neurologist in related settings. The primary care physician or internist can help to oversee the general care and communicate with family and with multiple specialists.

In addition to specialist physicians, help and support from various ancillary services go a long way in caring for the patient. They include physiotherapists who can help to ambulate and exercise the patients, pulmonary technicians who manage the ventilators and give chest physiotherapy, nutritionists who can oversee the oral and parenteral feeding, discharge coordinators and home health specialists who can help with postsurgical care. Nursing staff in the operating room and on the floors are extremely important members of the team. They also include nurse anesthetists [Certified Registered Nurse Anesthetist (CRNA)], physician assistants (PA), and nurse practitioners. A patient sees them more often than the doctors and asks for clarifications on various treatment protocols. Many of the new gadgets, both implantable and otherwise, need help from industry representatives who are specifically trained on the products or equipment. In their daily busy schedule, very often, surgeons forget to recognize the services rendered by these team members.

One negative aspect is fragmentation of health care with multiple interventionists and specialists doing bits and pieces of patient management. The surgeon should remain in charge of the patient as a common thread if the underlying pathology is a surgical disorder, even if the treatment or intervention is rendered by a different specialist.

KEY POINTS

Consultants can help the surgeon from carrying the burden of total care and responsibility. A better patient outcome is possible with teamwork and the surgeon can focus on the technical conduct of the surgical procedure. In fact, failure to obtain an appropriate consultation in a timely fashion can result in liability issues.

CHAPTER 82

Surgical Challenge Situations

INTRODUCTION

Surgeons are likely to be faced with difficult and challenging situations from time to time. It used to be said that the abdomen is a "pandora's box," implying that one would never know what they will find, and instant decision had to be made with an open abdomen. With the advent of modern imaging technology and minimally invasive procedures, such situations can be better anticipated and avoided. Still every surgeon will encounter some challenges in their career. Some such examples are given here.

PROBLEM APPENDIX

During surgery for appendicitis, one is unable to find the appendix: Mobilize the cecum completely from the terminal ileum to mid ascending colon. Follow the tinea on the cecum down to its very end at the bottom of the bulb. Look behind the cecum and ascending colon for a retrocecal appendix, adherent to the back wall of it. Slowly dissect it out from the colonic wall. It may not have the usual free mesoappendix.

Another possibility is that the appendix had been removed in the past during some other procedure as an incidental step. With the advent of laparoscopic procedures, incidental appendectomies occur with no separate incision. Look carefully for some other reasons for the current symptoms such as inflammatory bowel disease, mesenteric adenitis, tubo-ovarian pathology, pelvic inflammatory disease, inflammation of cecum due to parasitic infections, or even cancer of cecum.

Another scenario is that the appendix is appearing normal but one of the above mentioned reasons is the actual cause of pain and symptoms. Should one still do the appendectomy? If the base of the appendix is normal, one can still go ahead with the appendectomy to avoid future confusion and treat the underlying cause at the same time.

Another situation is incidental finding of Meckel's diverticulum during an emergency appendectomy. Should one do anything about it? Proper action is to do only the appendectomy and nothing else at that time.

Postoperatively, the pathology report comes back as showing evidence of adenocarcinoma or carcinoid in the appendix. What should one do? If it is adenocarcinoma of the appendix, one should do a proper right hemicolectomy for cancer clearance after staging and oncology consult. If the carcinoid is very small at the tip of the appendix, with the base being free of any involvement, it would be acceptable to do no further surgery, but follow with staging and oncology follow-up.

If one finds a cecal tumor instead of appendicitis, it would be best to do a right hemicolectomy at the same sitting. Antibiotics are given intravenously. A primary ileocolic anastomosis can be done without bowel preparation.

Is an incidental appendectomy justified when doing some other procedure intra-abdominally? The author is against doing any type of incidental and unplanned procedures.

PROBLEM HERNIA

Besides unexpected injuries to vas deferens, testicular artery, and iliac vessels, one may encounter decision-making situations.

If one finds unexpected presence of appendix in the hernial sac, should an appendectomy be done as it is easily visible and accessible? The author is against any incidental procedures. Same goes for the incidental finding of Meckel's diverticulum in the hernial sac.

If one finds metastatic cancer nodule in the hernial sac? The patient must be further investigated to find the primary and follow-up cancer care should be rendered. In all probability, this patient has widespread intra-abdominal metastasis.

If one is operating on a strangulated inguinal or femoral hernia, it is better to prepare and drape for a laparotomy and groin hernia repair together. If a strangulated segment of bowel is found which is not easily reducible or if it looks ischemic, immediate lower midline laparotomy should be performed. Care is taken to avoid perforation of the bowel during reduction. Very carefully, the hernial defect is widened using blunt forceps, and the bowel is gently pushed and pulled from inside and outside. Once the air bubble caught in the bowel is released internally, the bowel will shrink and reduce. After reduction, the involved bowel segment is covered with wet warm lap pads and kept immersed in warm saline irrigation fluid. It needs to be observed for few minutes. This time is used to repair the hernial defect, and the hernia part of surgery can be completed. The involved bowel segment is reinspected. At times, there is complete recovery with good mesenteric pulsation, in which case, it can be left alone. If there is any question about vascularity of the bowel, then immediate resection with end-to-end anastomosis is done.

PROBLEM GALLBLADDER

Gallbladder cannot be found at surgery: It is possible that it is an intrahepatic gallbladder or it is a very small shrunken gallbladder with a solitary stone inside. Careful dissection of the porta hepatis and intraoperative ultrasound are helpful. It is also possible that it had been removed prior to surgery.

Very difficult inflamed gallbladder: Steps that will help are: Decompress the fundus to remove the bile. Do not hesitate to convert from laparoscopic to open procedure. Dissect from fundus down. Open the gallbladder and remove all the stones. Stop with a subtotal cholecystectomy. Do a cholecystogram on the table to find the anatomy. Drain the liver bed before closing.

Postcholecystectomy severe abdominal pain: Suspect bile leak. Computed tomography (CT) scan will show subhepatic fluid collection. Percutaneous drainage of the area under CT guidance by interventional radiology will confirm bile leak. Urgent endoscopic retrograde cholangiopancreatography (ERCP) and stent placement across the common bile duct will help to heal the leak, especially if it is only a cystic duct leak. If major bile duct injury is noted, consider referral to a tertiary care center or perform open surgical repair.

DECISION TO DIVERT BOWEL

When to add a colostomy or ileostomy to an otherwise planned bowel surgery? One situation is to protect a very low rectal anastomosis that was done under tenuous conditions. Another situation is to divert first and wait for several days before a more definitive procedure. This would include an obstructing cancer of rectum, severely distended colon from megacolon or volvulus, perforated acute diverticulitis, and injury to mid-rectum. Toxic megacolon secondary to *Clostridium difficile* infection usually requires subtotal colectomy with ileorectal anastomosis, but another option is do diverting ileostomy, lavage of the colon, and wait for the megacolon to settle down. Following abdominoperineal resection for carcinoma of rectum, a permanent colostomy is inevitable. Following total colectomy for severe ulcerative colitis, a permanent ileostomy is necessary. Severe perineal infections with nonhealing wounds and watering-can perineum with multiple fistulae are other reasons to consider colostomy.

OCCULT PRIMARY

A metastatic deposit is noted but the primary is still unknown: This becomes a challenge. Often it is an enlarged lymph node that shows metastatic carcinoma. A careful evaluation and workup is needed.

If it is the cervical lymph node that is involved, often the primary is in the hidden parts of the head and neck. Hypopharynx, nasopharynx, and oropharynx are thoroughly checked with the help of ear, nose, and throat (ENT) consultants to include endoscopic evaluations. CT scan and magnetic resonance imaging (MRI) of the head and neck are done. Sinuses of the head area, thyroid, and scalp are other areas to look for. Melanomas can disappear or look like keratotic areas on the scalp. Virchow's lymph nodes are in the supraclavicular area from the primary in the abdominal viscera or testicle.

If the involved lymph node is in the axilla, the breast would be suspect. Mammogram and, if necessary, MRI of the breast are done and suspicious areas biopsied. Another possibility is a lesion in the upper extremity or front or back of the chest wall.

If it is in the groin area, one would look for lesions in the scrotum, penis, anal area, entire lower extremity, lower back and abdominal wall, and gluteal area.

Computed tomography scan shows an abnormal deposit on the liver, which on needle biopsy reveals it to be metastatic deposit. Primary is still unknown. One will have to do a complete gastrointestinal (GI) workup to include upper and lower endoscopies. Pancreas needs evaluation as it is an asymptomatic cancer in the initial phase. Similarly, CT scan of chest can show multiple metastatic deposits in the lung fields before primary makes itself evident.

Discussion ensues as to whether one should treat the metastatic lymph nodes with radical lymph node dissection any way, even when primary has not been detected.

In certain instances, the primary may not be resectable and may be better treated by radiation and chemotherapy.

A multidisciplinary tumor board meeting with participation by pathologist, radiation therapist, oncologist, and surgeon will help to sort out cases on an individual basis.

KEY POINTS

Surgeon can face challenges in making correct decisions, either in elective cases or in emergency situations and even in the operating room on the spot. Careful and systematic approach will help to solve them.

Chapter 83: Wellness

INTRODUCTION

Advising patients on healthy habits and wellness measures is a part of good medicine. Surgery is just one of the methods of getting them well and it is mostly a one-time intervention. Both preoperatively and postoperatively, they have to follow guidelines on maintenance of good health. It is like repairing a car or a machine. Surgery is similar to a one-time major repair. But regular maintenance is what is going to help that repair last long.

From prehistoric times, generations of people all over the world have wanted to live longer and healthier lives. The search for a youth potion, immortality, and perpetual good life is sought in every religion and epic stories. So, it is of no wonder that patients ask for advice to prevent heart attack, stroke, and to have a healthy life. Much of the discussion is good for prevention of atherosclerosis, falls, depression, and dementia, in addition to cancer screening as described in a previous chapter.

DIET

A Mediterranean diet is considered one of the best examples of a good diet. It consists of vegetables, lentils, beans, rice, nuts, fruits, fish, or fish oil supplements. It is best to avoid fatty and greasy food, sugary stuff, cola drinks, animal fat, and red meat. Processed food, trans fat, and fried food and snacks are avoided. Quantity should be controlled to avoid obesity. Calorie count is checked to avoid excessive calories per day.

EXERCISE

Daily exercise of any type is very helpful to maintain joint flexibility and muscle strength. It reduces obesity and reduces atherosclerosis build-up. Exercise helps to reduce cancers and dementia. Ambulation helps to reduce deep vein thrombosis, improves muscle strength, reduces falls due to improved balancing, and allows faster recovery from surgery. Simple walking for 30 minutes a day would be adequate. Group activities and sports will bring more fun and enjoyment.

STRESS REDUCTION

Any method to reduce stress, anxiety, and isolation is useful to reduce the onset of mental depression and inaction. Family, social activities, friends, group activities of any kind, visiting places of worship, meditation, and yoga are all of use.

MENTAL WORK

Keeping the brain engaged will reduce the onset of dementia and will help new neuronal sprouts. This can be in any way, including playing brain games, reading, writing, teaching, arts and crafts, and working.

ADDICTIVE HABITS

- Avoidance of certain addictive habits such as smoking, chewing tobacco, snuffing, and excess use of alcohol
- Avoidance of addictive prescription drugs, narcotic analgesics, such as Percocet® and OxyContin®
- Avoidance of addictive illegal drugs, such as cocaine, heroin, and synthetic drugs.

DENTAL HYGIENE

Routine dental care gets less attention in many third-world countries. Good dental hygiene prevents many oral cavity problems as well as systemic problems. It also improves social interactions and self-confidence.

SAFETY

Prevention of accidents, injuries, and falls is critical. Many surgical procedures and following side effects can be avoided by being careful. They also include avoiding pollutions of various types from air, water, food, and noise. Safe sex and use of condoms can prevent sexually transmitted diseases.

Good hygienic habits, including dental care, hand washing, and sanitation precautions, are equally important.

MEDICATIONS AND DISEASE MANAGEMENT

Control of known chronic medical conditions such as diabetes mellitus, hypertension, respiratory problems, allergic conditions, neurological, or urological problems with proper medical checkup, medications, and follow-up reduces their side effects.

Sleep

At least 7-8 hours of good sleep is recommended for all. Inadequate sleep can lead to poor health, errors, stress, obesity and irritability. Surgeons are at risk for the aftereffects of sleeplessness due to their unpredictable work schedule.

Peace and Happiness

Efforts must be made to find acceptance, peace, and happiness in life. It may be in the form of prayer, meditation, volunteer work, family, socialization, nature, music, or art. Good health needs both mental and physical well-being.

KEY POINTS

Health and wellness tips come in handy when talking to patients for whatever reason. They are applicable for all postoperative care and will lead to further betterment.

CHAPTER 84

Sign-out and Transfers

INTRODUCTION

A chain is strong only when the links are held together. In other words, one link is enough to break an entire chain. That is how the healthcare system works today. Many times, during the day, patient care is handed over to another healthcare provider. If both parties do not work with due diligence, many things can fall through the cracks, resulting in a delay of treatment or causing adverse outcomes.

MANAGEMENT

In daily hospital practice, it will be necessary to sign out or transfer care to others for various reasons. No one can work for 24 hours, 7 days a week, continuously. House physicians and junior physicians take calls and rotations all the time. Patients are frequently transferred from one location of the hospital to another location for various reasons. Much of the communication breakdown and "fall in the crack" occurs during this hand-off period. It is imperative to have hospital protocols and physician and nursing awareness to minimize patient disruption and to ensure continuity in these situations.

Emergency room to hospital room, regular room to intensive care or special units, floor rooms to operating rooms, operating room to recovery units, recovery room to regular floors or to intensive care units; change of shifts, call schedules, change in assignment of duties, rotation of doctors to different departments or units, transfer of doctors to different hospitals; family vacations and medical or sick leave are all various occasions when sign-off within the hospital is required.

A transfer from one hospital to another hospital may be required at times. This could be because of family requests, insurance, or financial reasons. Sometimes they have to be sent to advanced care centers for the management of complex issues. Sometimes it is to a lower-level facility for prolonged care such as rehabilitation and nursing care.

During the sign-out, if possible, both parties should participate in a direct conversation followed by a written communication. A physician-to-physician conversation between the discharging physician and accepting physician should be documented. All relevant details of the patient's history, physical examination findings, test results, presumptive diagnosis, treatment plans, and future plans must be discussed. Orders written as well as treatments, completed and uncompleted, should be pointed out. Preferably, the sign-out note as well as a sign-in note should be written in the chart, especially if the treating doctor is not going to be reachable for questions later on. A new set of entire orders should be written when the patient is in the hands of a new doctor or in a new location.

KEY POINTS

Errors and breakdown in communication can occur if willful efforts are not undertaken to avoid the same. One common area of such breakdown occurs when there is hand-off between providers or between areas of service inside the hospital.

CHAPTER 85

Safety in Surgery

INTRODUCTION

Do no harm. In other words, the treatment should not be worse than the disease. It is of paramount importance to conduct the surgery safely and minimize the complications and errors.

SAFETY AND QUALITY

Safety is conducting an activity with the least mistakes and errors—"being safe." Quality, on the other hand, is improving the standards and finding a better way of doing the work with better outcome. Safety and quality go hand in hand.

The Surgical Care Improvement Project (SCIP) was introduced for this purpose. They include measures to reduce surgical site infections, time-out or checklists, deep vein thrombosis (DVT) prophylaxis, appropriate use of antibiotics, allergy alerts, removal of catheters and intravenous (IV) lines in a timely fashion, documentation and communication, use of electronic medical records, preoperative evaluation of risk factors, maintaining sterile instruments and sterile techniques by all personnel, use of personal protective equipment (PPE), avoiding fire and energy hazards in the operating room, reducing anesthesia hazards, postoperative checklists, temperature regulation, glucose monitoring, nutritional support, prevention of falls, and beta-blocker therapy when indicated.

Checklists or time-out measures are well-accepted protocols now. The steps start from the doctor's office itself. Identifying risk factors, correcting laboratory abnormalities before surgery, stopping anticoagulants and antiplatelet agents, arranging for blood transfusion if necessary, treating medical conditions to optimize surgical risk, obtaining cardiac or pulmonary evaluations, obtaining informed consent and preparing correct documents with history and physical examination findings are all part of it. All team members, from anesthesia, nursing, assistants, and surgeon should participate in the checklists. They are done in the holding area before taking the patient to the operating room and the surgeon marks the site of incision. After induction of anesthesia, before the incision is made, patient identification, type of surgery, and consent are recited. After the main procedure, the instrument and sponge count are done to avoid leftover foreign bodies. After the surgery, lessons learned and problems encountered are analyzed and specimens are marked correctly for pathology examinations.

Some of these measures have already been discussed under various chapters in this book. Safety and quality measures are mandated by the Center for Medicare Services (CMS). It is proven by statistics that safety and quality measures improve patient outcome and reduce chances for medical malpractice claims.

Safety also implies technical safety in conducting proposed surgery. The best way to do a procedure is the way the surgeon is most comfortable in doing it. There is much competition and peer pressure forcing one to try new devices and new options. The surgeon should have adequate familiarity and training in adopting these methods. When the laparoscopic cholecystectomy was first introduced, there were many cases of bile duct injuries. It took a few years of training to know the importance of "clear view dissection" of the bile duct cystic artery and cystic duct. At times, patient's condition demands a less invasive or minimally invasive procedure. It is safer for that patient. It is safer to have a competent assistant or another surgeon to help in a complex operation than trying to do it solo. Surgeons should minimize operating time, especially doing open abdominal surgery. At the same time, hurrying up an operation is not good either. The surgeon should know the exact anatomy of blood vessels in order to control the vessels before incising into those areas. The same precautions go for avoiding nerve injuries and ureteric injuries. Surgery should be limited to do only what was intended to be done. It is best to avoid any type of incidental procedures.

Fire in the operating room is a real danger since inflammable energy devices are being used near oxygen. Internal injuries inadvertently can occur during laparoscopic procedures, while using energy devices, since they can occur outside of the visual field. Smoke inhalation from cautery and lasers can cause health issues and smoke evacuators are used. Leftover foreign bodies are real and happens despite needle and sponge counts. Surgeons can help by the regular habit of handing over needles on the needle holder and using only the necessary number of lap pads and sponges inside the field. Writing information visibly on a chalkboard can help with time, steps, personnel, counts, etc. Distractions lead to attention deficit and errors. They include loud music, frequent visitors, use of mobile phones, frequent change of team members, tired and sleepless or burnt-out surgeon and staff, unnecessary loud conversations during the procedure, lack of supplies, and time spent on documentation on computer.

Safety measures are combined with hospital risk management policies and quality improvement protocols. Sentinel events are adverse events which could result in negative outcome. Such events are studied for corrective action by changing the protocols, staffing, education, and training. The Hospital Quality Improvement Committee (QI Committee) and Joint Commission for Accreditation of Hospitals (JCAHO) are involved in such quality improvement measures. Root cause analysis and corrective steps and follow-up on the corrective steps are the goals instead of blame and shame on individuals.

It is possible that artificial intelligence technology will be used in the future to make analyses and predictions. In the US healthcare system, there is already an attempt to incentivize value-based reimbursement. In other words, quality of care rendered by the physician could be tied to the reimbursement of fee.

KEY POINTS

Safety of the patient and avoiding errors are very important. Having a routine system and team participation can help accomplish this.

Medical Malpractice Concerns

INTRODUCTION

Patients and families feel disappointed and disheartened when there is an adverse outcome, particularly when they feel the physician and hospital did not follow community standards, when there is a cover-up, and when there is a lack of caring and empathy. Their reaction could be filing a malpractice suit. In some areas of the world, they may take the law in their own hands and physically punish those whom they see as culprits.

MANAGEMENT

This is a civil suit filed by an aggrieved patient or family when the outcome goes wrong and results in damage or death. The rate of medical malpractice is very high in countries such as the United States of America and very low in certain African countries.

To prove a medical malpractice, there must be an error, there must be a consequential damage, and there must be a proof of negligence that caused the error. Negligence is based on community standards to some extent. How another physician of similar specialty would have handled the case under similar circumstances is used as a guideline.

As medical science progresses, the standard of treatment changes. For example, 100 years ago, many tests, drugs, and antibiotics were not available. Hence, many diagnostic errors or complications following surgeries that were occurring previously are now preventable.

Patient and family expectations and their perceptions also contribute to dissatisfaction. If they felt a lack of empathy or caring behavior by the healthcare providers, such types of impersonal attitudes can lead to confrontation. Communications, documentation, prompt and timely service, and competent care are the pillars that protect the physician against malpractice.

Physicians should know their limitations due to available facilities, staffing, and their own level of knowledge and skills. Instead of taking risks, it is better to transfer complex cases to referral hospitals or to specialist surgeons early on.

Certain types of errors are considered as "never ever" occurrences where society has adopted a zero tolerance. Such errors are operating on the wrong patient, wrong body part, wrong side of the body, or wrong operation. System protocols of the hospital and strict adherence to such protocols by all healthcare providers can reduce such adverse events. This includes identification of patients with wristbands, charts that go with the patient, checking identification of the patient by each and every provider before starting any treatment or intervention, and marking the site and side of surgery by the surgeon before taking the patient to the operating room. A "time out" is called just before the incision is made with participation of all members of the operating team, at which time, the name of the patient, diagnosis, type of surgery planned, side and site, instruments, and drugs are recited and agreed by all.

Leftover foreign bodies in the patient following surgery is another event that speaks for itself. These include needles, instruments, sponges, lap pads, and other objects used during surgery. They could be forgotten to be removed or lost. A classic situation is a lap pad that has been used to pack away bowels or to stop bleeding in the pelvis or in the subphrenic regions. Therefore, a count of all instruments, lap pads, and needles is made before surgery and after completion of the main surgery, but before closing the abdomen.

Complications and mishaps are bound to happen since no one is perfect in life. However, efforts must be made to avoid them by following community standards. As soon as such an adverse event occurs, it should be recognized, corrected, and remedial measures undertaken. The patient

> **BOX 86.1:** Avoiding medical malpractice.
>
> - Practice evidence-based medicine, do the right thing
> - Communicate and communicate with everyone
> - Document and document
> - Be a master in your field
> - Safety of the patient comes first
> - Show empathy and caring
> - Accept the errors and take immediate corrective steps
> - Obtain tests and consultations as necessary
> - Do not falsify records or cover up—they will backfire

and family must be informed about the adverse events and follow-up care planned.

KEY POINTS

The practice of good medicine is by being a master in the field of work, providing competent and timely care, good communication and documentation, and showing empathy and caring attitude—these are the ways to avoid medical malpractice suits **(Box 86.1)**.

EU GSPR Authorised Reprsentative
Logos Europe, 9 rue Nicolas Poussin
1700, La Rochelle, France
Phone: +33 (0) 6 67 93 73 78
E-mail: contact@logoseurope.eu

www.ingramcontent.com/pod-product-compliance
Ingram Content Group UK Ltd.
Pitfield, Milton Keynes, MK11 3LW, UK
UKHW050458150426